To Hell and Back

To Hell and Back

Humans of COVID

Barkha Dutt

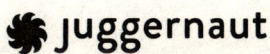

JUGGERNAUT BOOKS
C-I-128, First Floor, Sangam Vihar, Near Holi Chowk,
New Delhi 110080, India

First published by Juggernaut Books 2022

Copyright © Barkha Dutt 2022

10 9 8 7 6 5 4 3 2 1

P-ISBN: 9789391165574
E-ISBN: 9789391165659

The views and opinions expressed in this book are the author's own. The facts contained herein were reported to be true as on the date of publication by the author to the publishers of the book, and the publishers are not in any way liable for their accuracy or veracity.

All rights reserved. No part of this publication may be reproduced, transmitted, or stored in a retrieval system in any form or by any means without the written permission of the publisher.

Typeset in Adobe Caslon Pro by R. Ajith Kumar, Noida

Printed at Thomson Press India Ltd

For Speedy Dutt,
extraordinary father, kindest friend, brightest mind,
generous heart and noble soul.

And for all of you who trusted me to tell your story.

Dear Rehaan
lots of love
hope you like it.

Barkha Dutt

Contents

1. The Village with the Yellow Water — 3
2. The Exodus — 19
3. The First Responders — 51
4. Five Girls and a Funeral — 77
5. Leelawati and the Loneliness of the Elderly — 97
6. 'Nobody Teaches You this at Harvard' — 107
7. 'They have Blood on Their Hands' — 125
8. Fathers and Daughters — 141
9. Asphyxiated — 161
10. *'Awaaz De Kahan Hai'* — 185
11. The COVID Pallbearers — 209
12. The Children of COVID — 227
13. And Then Came Omicron — 249

Notes — 263
Acknowledgements — 267

In early 2020, as India entered the world's largest lockdown in response to the first wave of COVID, I left my home with a small team of three, packed into a Maruti Ertiga, on a journey that would take us across the length and breadth of the country. We travelled from Delhi in the north, to Kerala in the south, back to Ladakh in the Himalayas, covering 30,000 kilometres, quite literally on the road with the pandemic.

During the ferocious and devastating second wave in 2021, we were back on the ground – in the hinterland, remote rural interiors and along the banks of the Ganga where hundreds of bodies had washed ashore or been buried in the sand.

In 2022, as the Omicron wave sweeps through India, we are once again travelling to chronicle the consequences of the virus on our schools, hospitals and social structures. The reportage of COVID has taken up all of my life over two years, and now counting.

This book is about all that we saw and have learnt. It is about people, not numbers. It is rooted in extensive ground reportage, but it is also deeply personal. It is partly about me, but it is mostly about our country.

It is about all those who suffered and struggled, lost and loved.

It is about the humans of COVID.

1

The Village with the Yellow Water

Somewhere along National Highway 44, the longest stretch of road in India connecting Kashmir in the north to Kanyakumari at the southernmost end of the country, lies the village of Kundli, in the district of Sonipat in Haryana.

An industrial township has been built all around the village, with smoke-spewing manufacturing units that produce processed food items, leather, garments and accessories.

For Sonipat, no more than an hour from Delhi, where there were once only open wheat fields and roadside dhabas serving parathas with blobs of white butter and greasy pickle, the industrial zone was a major development milestone.

The village itself hasn't changed much in years, despite sitting in the lap of these factories.

In the first week of April 2020, when the world's hazy and still incorrect understanding of COVID was that the virus jumped from surface to surface – in what is called fomite transmission – I made a trip to Kundli. At this time, the guidance from the World Health Organization (WHO) was to wash hands frequently as one way to remain safe in the pandemic. Even after scientists discovered that the coronavirus rarely spreads because of contaminated surfaces and is mostly airborne in closed, unventilated areas, hand washing and sanitizing have remained part of the advisory guidelines.

In Kundli that afternoon, women had queued up at the main water line to fill their buckets and bottles and carry them home. It is estimated that women across India spend 150 million work days every year fetching and carrying water.[1]

Kundli village was no different: here too this burden fell on the women.

But the water that trickled out of the tap was urine-yellow in colour.

'*Yeh paani hai ji, yahan ka, yeh Kundli gaon ka paani hai,*' (This is the water of Kundli village) said Manju, pointing to the plastic container that was once a can of paint and was now filled to the brim with an oily chemical. This was the water her village got.

Then, pulling back the sleeves of her kurta, she pointed to the rashes all along her arm. They were down her back too. 'This is what happens to us from bathing with this water.' Industrial waste had contaminated and corroded the underground soil. The water was not just undrinkable, it was entirely unusable, even for the simple purpose of keeping hands clean during a pandemic. Residents of the village came forward one by one, presenting bottles and pots of water that looked more like cheap cooking oil. Then they showed us scabs, rashes and wounds, and described a host of other allergies that the toxic water had caused.

What did they do for drinking water, I wondered. 'We usually have to spend ten rupees to buy a jug of filtered water,' lamented Manju.

But ever since the midnight of 24 March 2020, when a nationwide lockdown was enforced to contain the spread of

COVID, all economic activity had come to an abrupt halt here. Those living on subsistence daily wages found forking out cash for water even tougher.

The village with the yellow water was an early lesson for me in what would become my overarching learning from reporting COVID from across India, through 2020 and 2021 – the virus was anything but the great equalizer. It exacerbated existing inequalities and birthed new ones. In an already stratified society, it created a new social order. The assumption that the calamity was inherently egalitarian – that the pandemic had somehow created a level playing field on which death and illness were the great levellers, flattening out the ground for India's wealthiest and poorest – was grossly incorrect.

Yes, it's true that almost no Indian in a country of 1.3 billion has been left untouched over the two seasons of sadness, and there could yet be more suffering ahead. We have all either lost someone we love, had bouts of severe illness, lost jobs and incomes, struggled to keep our businesses afloat, helplessly watched our children drop out of school or fall back in learning, or wrestled with loneliness, alienation and social dysfunction. And grief does have a sledgehammer way of hollowing out the heart, no matter whether you are a CEO or a clerk. But the way those who live at the margins of power and economic access experienced the horrors of COVID is incomparable with the travails of the more privileged.

On the banks of the Yamuna river, looking out at the swanky, eight-lane Delhi–Noida Direct (DND) expressway is the village of Chilla Khadar. It was in April 2020, again, while reporting on the initial aftermath of the lockdown, that I discovered you could only get to it by boat. Once you dropped off the swish city roads, just ahead of Delhi's border with Uttar Pradesh, and wove past sparsely populated villages, the dust tracks opened up to a riverbank. Here a handful of fisherfolk sat by the water, their blue nets spread over a few wooden boats. We clambered on to one and our boatman rowed us on the placid waters, past clusters of green shoots of patera (*Dicliptera*) growing all around, to the tiny settlement in India's capital that still had no road access. Many residents here made a living by selling these shoots in the wholesale mandis to shopkeepers, who in turn used the plant's natural threads to tie together clumps of spinach, okra or beans. Their other source of daily income was to catch fish for contractors who had a licence to do so from the Delhi government. They would get a fixed daily wage for their labour. With the lockdown in place, both sources of earning were entirely frozen.

On the other side of the river, a small pathway through a forested cover led us to a collection of huts. Some were just made from plastic sheets thrown over thatch and bamboo. About eighty to one hundred people, men and women, were sitting out in the open. Their already tough lives had been compounded by the lockdown. 'Our ration, our doctors, our schools . . . everything has to be done by boat,' said Susheela. 'How do we eat? Where do we go for work?'

Just earlier that year the National Human Rights Commission had taken note of the fact that the children of Chilla Khadar were risking their lives to get to school. Every morning, a small group of twenty kids would first cover a 250-metre distance on the river by boat; then they would link arms and walk up a steep slope, through brambles and over fences, to reach the nearest government-run school which was half an hour's walk away.

I thought of COVID and wondered how an ambulance would reach a patient in distress here.

'Even if someone has a heart attack here, he has to be taken by boat to the nearest point along the Yamuna plain, just by the temple. There he is placed on a hand cart used by vegetable vendors and taken to the nearest hospital,' said Som Bhai, a grassroots activist who had spent years advocating for the village.

In Mumbai, where Dharavi, Asia's biggest slum, had emerged as a COVID red zone, I spent some time outside a community toilet to discover that the pandemic slogans of hygiene and hand washing had literally no meaning in an area where 8,000 common toilets were used by over 850,000 people.

On the wall outside one of the common toilets, a visual manifestation of the virus had been painted as a mural across the breadth of the washroom. Imagined as a hydra-headed, bright-eyed green monster with its tongue cheekily sticking out, it looked oddly friendly and familial, a sort of homely, amiable ghost.

But containing COVID in Dharavi where 850,000 people were packed into a 2.4-square-kilometre area, making it one of the most densely populated areas of the world, was a nightmare. And that hundreds of people, men, women and children, used common bathroom stalls to bathe, urinate and defecate made it just that much more difficult.

The common toilets were really just a shack held up by wooden poles, the individual toilets separated by walls. At one set of toilets, a young boy stood at the entrance, indifferently collecting money before he let people in, women to the right, men to the left. There were nine stalls on either side. On a small table outside a plastic bottle of water, a jar of soap and a sanitizer had been hastily added as an afterthought.

To come here was to realize the theoretical elitism of the pandemic public service advertisements. 'Stay at home' was the most common message of the lockdown months, often enforced by dogmatic police personnel. But what value did it possibly have in Dharavi, where anywhere between five and eight people lived cheek by jowl in confined, unventilated and tiny closed spaces?

It wasn't just in Dharavi that one found crowded homes in the country: 92 million households in India live in one room; another 78 million live in two-room homes.[2] The borrowed Western concept of pushing people indoors, given the average Indian family size of five, only underlined how the summers of 2020 and 2021 have been especially cruel for India's poor.

The pandemic has mercilessly uncovered all our gaps – in resources, healthcare, education, social structures – and yes, even in journalism.

One hundred and sixty million Indians do not have access to clean drinking water. Two hundred thousand Indians die every year from drinking unsafe water, and nearly 38 million fall ill from waterborne diseases annually. But in the newsrooms of mainstream media organizations, the story of Kundli and its corrosive water would have been mostly considered too 'soft' to be pursued by the top guns. Admittedly, before 2020, as a long-time conflict-and-war correspondent more accustomed to reporting on insurgencies rather than inequality, I would have felt the same. As a woman in the media who has had to work really hard to prove my 'toughness', my natural instinct all these years has been to shrug off assignments that could be slotted as 'features'. And so, I 'progressed' from on-ground reportage of calamity and chaos and riots and revolts to chasing politicians on prime time, because that is how the hierarchical ladder on which your career climbs has always been structured in our television networks and newspapers.

As a child of TV – I joined the industry when India's public broadcaster Doordarshan was the country's only channel, only just beginning 30-minute capsules of privately produced news bulletins – I have been moulded by the magic and immediacy of the visual medium. But I have also seen – and I must confess have been a participant in – the collapse of television news.

Broken revenue models, ballooning costs, shrinking budgets for travel and some twisted idea that shouty, contrarian guests make for great viewing reduced TV news to being talk-driven and made studio rats of so many of us. Though I would always try and retain my identity as a ground reporter and go to where the story is, I can't deny that over the years I too slowly got caught up in measuring my self-worth by how many 'important' people I could bring on to my shows. The domination of the studio made us increasingly lazy, stale, unimaginative and without empathy. It disconnected us from audiences and made our journalism more about celebrities and less about people.

By 24 March 2020, when Prime Minister Modi announced the decision to lock down India, as many other nations had done to fight COVID, I had finally given up on television. After quitting NDTV, a network where I worked for twenty-two years, and a couple of ill-conceived partnerships later, I was readying to build my own digital platform. We were tiny in contrast to the behemoths I had long been part of. Fewer than six people, we operated from a small office in the basement of my home.

But as COVID began sweeping through India and the world's largest lockdown was enforced, I knew that this was the biggest news story of my lifetime. Perhaps for the first time since 1999, when I had reported the Kargil war between India and Pakistan from the trenches, COVID was an assignment that kept me awake at night. In fact, in some ways I can bookend my two-decades-plus in journalism with these two definitive assignments of my professional life – Kargil in 1999 and COVID in 2020.

Like back then, now too I was plagued by restlessness. I knew I would not be able to rest in the safe, sanitized environs of a broadcast studio, chronicling the pandemic from behind a shiny sunmica set. After all, journalists were listed as an essential service, exempt from the curfew restrictions for a reason. This was a test like none other, of both calibre and commitment. To fail this moment would be to not have been a journalist at all.

From the very first morning after the lockdown, when I went to the borders of the capital and saw the beginnings of the great march of the country's migrant workers heading back to their homes on foot, I knew that this had to be chronicled from out there, from among the people. The humanitarian tragedy was the preamble to the medical crisis, and in some ways even dwarfed it at first.

And so, four of us clambered on to my Maruti Ertiga – Vinod, the valiant driver, my producer Prashanti, my cameraperson Madan and myself – and we began hitting the road. At first, we would drive to a motorable destination, spending anywhere between five and ten hours on the road, a couple of hours at the location, and head right back to Delhi. In the early weeks of the lockdown there was absolutely no food, water or place to stay available anywhere. We would pack small bags of biscuits and water and head out. Sometimes we would sleep in the car.

Then we realized that in order to report across the length and breadth of India and not be only north-centric, we would have to take the plunge and take our chances. And so began our journey, by road, across the country.

In over 120 days we covered 30,000 kilometres and fourteen

states and union territories, including a dramatic turnaround from the border of Bihar to Delhi to make our way to Ladakh, where in the middle of the pandemic a warlike situation was developing with China, where the virus had originated to begin with. When we first reached Mumbai by road, it felt like a small miracle; after that there was no holding us back. In Kerala we met Vishnu, a nurse on COVID duty who was also a Theyyam artiste. In Karnataka's Kalaburagi, we spoke to the family of India's first recorded victim who succumbed to COVID. In Kota, Rajasthan, our hearts broke for young students from Bihar stranded at coaching centres, enraged that their state wasn't ready to take them back home. In Patiala we marvelled at the stoicism of the police officer whose hand was cut off while trying to enforce the lockdown.

But the arc of our journey was shaped by the hundreds of thousands — and by the end of it, millions — of Indian citizens who had to walk back home.

The intimacy of strangers powered our travels. People we didn't know sent us home-cooked food. Those I had possibly just exchanged a single tweet with and possibly even been trolled by, opened up their homes. When my shoes split into two after weeks of wear and tear — remember, stores were closed — acquaintances sent new ones. When my car broke down my most vitriolic critics offered to drive us. Sometimes we'd get lucky and manage a hotel room. Some nights, we stayed in desolate guest houses with rats and cockroaches for company.

When the second wave of the virus announced itself, it was like Indian public health's 26/11 moment — and not only because it was a tectonic shift in how we see life and death or because of its generational trauma. In just the same way the 72-hour Mumbai siege by Pakistani terrorists brought terrorism home to the doors of the upper middle class and wealthy, 2021 brought the pandemic to the same lot, in a shift from the first year of the pandemic when mostly the poor had suffered. In its first year, the virus never created the level playing field the clichés suggested it would. If anything, it created a new social order of prejudice, as it wrenched open our fault lines to reveal a horrifically unequal country. When it became a People Like Us (PLU) pandemic in 2021, it brought people closer; but in some cases, it also triggered deep denial and a desperate need to look away from the calamity and its tactile sorrow. The pushback against cremation-ground reportage, for instance, by the supporters of the ruling BJP – I was called a vulture more times that I could count – was reminiscent of a similar reluctance to hear the voices of families whose relatives were trapped inside the Oberoi and Taj hotels during the Mumbai attack, even when they wished to tell their story.

It was almost as if 'unseeing' it would make it go away.

There was a similar attempt at erasing and obliterating the truth of the Ganga's graves.

India failed to save the living; now we were refusing to count our dead.

As election campaigns continued well into the third week of April in 2021, Shahid Jameel, one of the country's top virologists, told me: 'There will be many more mutations born from these mass gatherings,' breaking down in tears as he spoke of losing cousins to COVID. 'India has lost the plot.'

If 2020 held a mirror to our social inequities, 2021 broke the compact between citizen and state.

The intensity of the second act has unwittingly led to a slow erasure of the memory of the first. So we forget now that even in the first quarter of 2020 there was the suggestion that all India had to do was ride the wave till summer; the scorching tropical heat would take care of the rest. As the humanitarian crisis among the most marginalized Indians began to overshadow the medical emergency, one of India's top scientists wrote this message on 25 April 2020, to a closed group of friends on WhatsApp: 'Let's wait to see how it plays out. There is no evidence that summer heat or humidity will effect [sic] it. Until then it is speculation introduced by climate scientists. But I will say that this mockery of a lockdown is taking us deeper into the shit hole. Social factors, government high handedness and planning on the fly will ensure its failure. We should be mentally prepared to lose friends and relatives.'

By 25 April 2021, there was carnage.

This is a book about the people we met over our two years on the road covering the pandemic. It is about the Hindu gravedigger at a Muslim burial ground, about a Muslim volunteer who performed the last rites for a six-month-old Hindu baby, about the women in a housing society in Surat who decided to cook five rotis more at every meal to feed migrant workers in their city, about a nurse who found it easier to battle terrorists than COVID, about children who watched their mother die on the cold floor of a hospital after she was unable to get a bed in time, about young resident doctors and their mental meltdown, about children with autism and newborns infected with the virus, about gurudwaras that ran oxygen langars when hospitals closed their doors, about teachers who paid the price with their lives to keep our democracy functional in the middle of a pandemic, about the goodness and prejudice of ordinary people and about hope and heartbreak, mistakes and redemption, science and sentiment.

There are other, better books on the science of COVID, on

the policies that should or should not have been enforced, on the inside track of what the prime minister was thinking. This is not that book. This is about COVID's human story. About its victims, survivors and heroes. About its bereaved, bereft and brave. About a journey to hell and back.

For me, this is also personal.

For the past two years, my life had been consumed by COVID. As I travelled from the villages of Uttar Pradesh to the paddy fields of Kerala, from the mountains of Ladakh to the bastis of Mumbai, from the graves of the Ganga in Varanasi in which corpses floated, to documenting the pile-up of abandoned COVID bodies buried in the sandbanks of Prayagraj, one day, in April 2021, I became the news I was reporting.

My father died from COVID, and in the fight to get him an ICU bed, an ambulance, an oxygen cylinder – and later space at a crematorium – I literally became the same story I had chronicled. And on the day we cremated him, I tested positive for COVID.

In my twenty years of being a reporter I have often seen death and violence, loss and despair; I have seen bombs explode and bodies fragment. Because of my consistent exposure to conflict zones, I have learnt, over the years, to remain functional and efficient through the most inflammatory situations, at least while the news has to be captured on camera. I believed that consistent practice had given me the strength to absorb all that I witnessed.

But I found the writing of this book to be incredibly painful and difficult. I would often miss deadlines. I thought of abandoning it altogether more than once. I took a break from the daily cycle of news to spend a month in another country, thinking the peace and quiet would help me write. Instead, I found that I would cry inconsolably and without provocation, sometimes for hours on end. It was some sort of mental and emotional breakdown, a release perhaps of all that I had observed – and all that I had lost. All that we had lost, collectively.

I finally forced myself to complete the book, because if there is one thing that every single person I met on these travels had in common, it was this: no one wanted the people they loved to die uncounted, unsung, their stories unchronicled or untold.

As a mourner I met at a graveyard in Delhi said to me, 'Just because we are poor, it doesn't mean we have to die like insects, does it?'

On 30 January 2020, a third-year medical student from Wuhan University in China tested positive for COVID in Thrissur, Kerala. She was the first recorded case of COVID in India.

On 10 March, seventy-six-year-old Mohammed Hussein Sadiqi, who had recently returned from Saudi Arabia to Kalaburagi in Karnataka, died from COVID. His was the first official death from the virus.

At 8 p.m. on 24 March 2020, after a brief experiment with a fourteen-hour-long 'People's Curfew' two days earlier, Prime Minister Narendra Modi followed the global playbook on COVID with the announcement of a national lockdown. Shutting down 1.3 billion people made this the world's largest lockdown. But in a departure from what other countries had done, all public transport between states, including planes, trains and buses, was terminated. The lockdown came into play at midnight, giving the country just four hours' notice. Officials say the short window was deliberate so as to prevent widespread movement of people. The exact opposite happened. With all economic activity coming to a halt, millions of daily-wage workers left the cities of India for their villages on foot, walking hundreds of kilometres, with no food or water. In the first months of the pandemic, the humanitarian crisis overshadowed the medical threat of the virus.

2

The Exodus

On the outskirts of Delhi's city limits is Saraswati Kunj, an urban Haryana village tucked away in the forgotten shadow of shiny all-glass automobile centres and new-age fintech start-ups.

Dwarfed by high-rise luxury apartments named after flowers, hospitals that look like hotels with food courts and valet parking, and internet companies that have reimagined the idea of the office with technicolour beanbags, open-plan seating and coffee lounges, the slum quarter of Saraswati Kunj is an inconvenient reality check on the India story.

It is a barely memorable collection of shanties. Stray cows, hens let loose from their cages and three-legged wobbly street carts line the entrance to a slum where wooden poles hold up corrugated tin sheets in an approximation of residential rooms.

Shit, both animal and human, is piled up in the nallahs. The squalor is a way of life, barely noticeable to its residents.

Here, migrant workers live cheek by jowl, in a cul-de-sac that passes for a colony.

Mukesh Mandal was one such resident. He had migrated from Bihar, the eastern state with the second highest outflow of workers who left home in search of work, also the state famous for its distinctive Madhubani folk art – geometric patterns framing mythological figures, drawn using twigs, fingers and nib-brushes.

Mandal too was a painter.

He made a living working at houses in need of a facelift and the odd job at construction sites.

That morning, in April 2020, when we reached his home, the skies bellowed at the earth in a fit of grey and the rain turned the muddy pathways to Mandal's house into smelly slush. Mandal's wife Poonam was standing at the entrance, surrounded by a gaggle of children staring curiously and giggling nervously about what could have possibly brought visitors to their neighbourhood. Her face wore the tearless stains of extreme shock. With one arm she wordlessly held out a passport-size picture of her husband, urging us to take a closer look. Mandal's everyman face was framed by a goatee; he wore a pale-coloured shirt over a T-shirt. He was not smiling, not even for the photograph.

In the cradle of the other arm, Poonam balanced her youngest child, a scrawny infant with a runny nose, dressed in a sleeveless cotton frock, her hand pressed against her tiny mouth, as if to signal hunger. Poonam's dishevelled hair fell out in thin strands from under the yellow sari pallu that covered her head. She kept holding Mandal's ant-sized picture in the palm of her hand, saying nothing.

Her father, an elderly man with only one functional leg, hobbled forward with the help of a stick. The police had just left, he said, after interrogating the family.

Finding work and making ends meet had always been a challenge for Mukesh Mandal.

But since the midnight of 24 March, when Prime Minister

Narendra Modi took the decision to lock India down, all construction and commercial activity across the country had come to a halt. With that, so did Mandal's source of income.

Without subsistence wages, feeding a family of seven became instantly impossible.

India's national lockdown was initially meant to be in place for three weeks. It eventually lasted for over seventy days.

A non-governmental organization would come by every few days to distribute one-meal boxes; but it was far from enough. Mandal's four children were on the verge of starving.

The day before his death, Mandal had quietly left the house. He came back with ₹2,500. He kept ₹500 aside to purchase a table fan – temperatures had already hit the late thirties and there was no other ventilation inside their room. He handed the rest of the money to Poonam and told her to buy rice, dal and wheat.

When the family wondered how he had managed the money he revealed that he had pawned his mobile phone. '*Bhooke pyase mar jayenge.*' (We'll die of hunger.)

Those were his last words.

The next morning, while Poonam had stepped out to use the community bathroom shared by the slum dwellers, he took one of her dupattas, stepped into the empty quarter next to their room, tied it to the bamboo pole that gave support to the structure and took his life. He spoke to no one and left no suicide note. He was only thirty years old.

Mandal's father-in-law was at the temple down the road that morning. The police picked him up from there and led him to a mountain of paperwork. 'They ordered me to put my thumb on the documents,' said Dadaji, the sobriquet by which he is known locally. 'It's best for you to sign this and close it, otherwise you will be dragged into a long criminal case. You will be locked up,' the police warned. Dadaji was terrified. He can neither read nor write but he put his indigo-ink stamp of endorsement on whatever papers the cops thrust in his face.

The official closure report said Mandal's suicide was triggered by mental health problems. The local administration refused to take cognizance of the spectre of starvation that haunted Mukesh Mandal in his final hours.

His was one of the many lockdown deaths that will remain uncounted.

There is still no official data on how many might have been driven to death by suicide in the traumatic months of the lockdown. But between March and July 2020, the news media alone reported 419 such deaths in the country.

The lockdown upended economic supply chains across India. It also disrupted the public distribution system on which the abjectly poor depend for basic rations. In their first panicky avatar, instead of being an instrument to prevent large gatherings, the curbs on movement were essentially a police-enforced curfew. At a time when the Indian state should have shown its most benign, generous face, it ended up being intimidatory and draconian.

And you did not have to travel to remote interior villages or to the hinterland to discover that food was running short. Any settlement of migrant workers, even just on the outskirts of the capital, would tell the same story.

Past the 'English Beer and Wine Shops' and the cyber-tech parks were slums where most men and women were contract labour and street vendors. In a village not far from Mukesh Mandal's home, in Begumpur Khatola, almost all the residents were migrant labourers from Uttar Pradesh. They worked as contract employees in nearby factories or as small-time food hawkers. Those lucky enough to have monthly incomes had not received their salaries that month. And those suddenly stripped of daily wages found that they were unable to reach the government-run ration shops on foot. The farthest they could get without being turned back by the police was the neighbourhood gurudwara, from where they would load two puris and some sabzi to take back to feed their children.

India's finance minister had promised that 5 kilograms of wheat and 1 kilogram of rice per month would be available free of cost to each ration card holder in the public distribution system. But millions of workers had been forced out of the food security net, either because their ration cards had lapsed back in the village, or their applications for a card were still to be approved, or because they did not have Aadhaar cards or verifiable biometrics.

Under the shade of a peepal tree, across the street from the closed stores, was a small portrait of Ganesha placed next to an overturned, empty box of Dalda. On one of the downed shutters, an advertisement for Sufiyana Chai shared space with the smiling visage of Amitabh Bachchan, helpfully listing the health benefits of Emami vegetable oil. But there was no oil, tea, pulses or vegetables to be had here. Most of the residents said they had begun to borrow not just money but also grains and pulses from neighbours and relatives. One daily shared meal for the household was usually rice with dal or onion. Government-run shops that were mandated to supply free grains to those below the poverty line were either too far to be reached during a curfew or those in abject need did not have the required identity cards to procure them. By the Delhi government's estimate, India's capital alone had 2 million workers without ration cards.[3] Even this estimate was exceeded when close to 7 million people in Delhi applied for e-coupons to get dry rations under the government's special relief package without a ration card.⁴ A quick show of hands in Begumpur revealed almost no one had one. The safety net had come apart.

In the first two months of the lockdown, two states disbursed zero foodgrains and eleven distributed less than 1 per cent of the allocated foodgrains.⁵

India's poorest feared that hunger would kill them well before the virus did.

And they were not wrong.

Seventy-four per cent of migrant households confirmed that they had to significantly reduce the quantity of food they were eating in the first two months of the lockdown; 31 per cent of homes said they did not receive any free rations.⁶

And an overwhelming majority of the migrants decided that they simply could not take the chance to remain where they were.

On the eight-lane Yamuna Expressway, built at a cost of $1.8 billion (about ₹13,000 crores), stretching across a length of 165 kilometres, and linking Delhi to the City of Love, Agra, Ranveer Singh, thirty-eight, set out for home, on foot.

It was the morning of 27 March 2020, a Saturday. Ranveer worked as a delivery agent at Khana Khazana in Tughlakabad Extension, an assortment of illegally built narrow structures staring at a skyline of exposed electricity cables. He supervised the home delivery of greasy paneer bhurji, chicken saagwala and chicken 'lolypop', rolled into newspaper scrap and packed into white plastic bags, for which he was paid ₹10,000 every month.

Home was on the outskirts of Ambaha, in Morena district of Madhya Pradesh, past the Chambal ravines, the denuded riverbanks once known for dacoits as well as the seventeenth-century Sabalgarh fort, carved out of a giant rock face. He'd have to cross the borders of two states, Uttar Pradesh and Rajasthan, before the extravaganza of the highways would make way for dusty, pot-holed, rickety tracks, partly unbuilt and partly undone by wear and tear.

Back home, his wife Mamata pulled the corner of her synthetic blue sari more tightly over her head, as she sat hunched over on a collapsible cot in the open courtyard of their one-room house, paralysed with fear. Aradhya, all of three years old and the youngest of their three children, limped across the hot stone floor surface; she'd been born with a disability. Mamata wondered how she would look after her children if something were to happen to Ranveer.

Ranveer's sister, Pinki, a teacher at the village's Shanti Niketan Secondary School, leapt for the phone in hopeful anticipation when it rang that night at 8.23 p.m. She made a mental note of the precise turn of the clock as that familiar number flashed on her screen. One of the reasons that her brother had to move to the city was to repay the loan he had taken to get her married. That responsibility haunted her today. He still owed lenders ₹250,000. Subsisting on the ₹2,000 a month he earned, helping her out at the local school was impossible. Ranveer knew he would have to move to the city.

'*Paagal ho gaye ho kya?*' (Have you gone mad?) their elder brother shouted into the phone, as the family gathered around its crackly speaker. When Ranveer rang he was already 50 kilometres outside Delhi; he planned to cover the entire 308.5-kilometre-distance on foot. 'Just stay there, just stay where you are,' Pinki implored him.

But Ranveer walked, all by himself, past men and women and children who, just like him, walked in the hope of a homecoming.

Cement workers, potato farmers, construction labourers, hotel helps, diamond cutters, blanket weavers, factory supervisors – they walked under the blazing sun and through desolate, dark, moonless nights, sometimes barefoot and sometimes wearing flip-flop slippers made from rubber, their entire universe tied into small sacks carried aloft on their shoulders, holding on to the last packet of glucose biscuits and water before those too ran out. The women carried the physical belongings, stuffed usually into a makeshift carry bag knotted from a spare sari; the men carried their toddlers on their backs.

Yet, for almost two months, at least 100 million internal migrants, among the country's poorest citizens, who moved from the villages to the cities in search of work, either seasonally or semi-permanently, remained on the margins of political, public and media attention.[7] They were India's invisible people. This was the glaring ethical crater in the world's largest lockdown. The virus that was supposed to subsume all our differences did anything but. It held a mirror to our stratified, hierarchical society; it pulled at us to look at our reflection, to confront our pockmarked truth and concede our horrifying inequities, even as we desperately tried to look the other way.

The sealed borders of India's states became battlegrounds, testing the will, the resilience and the fighting capacity of millions of its citizens.

On 29 March, a day after Ranveer Singh had embarked on his expedition home and a full five days after the country had been put under lock and key, the government issued its first diktat on wages. Signed by the Indian home secretary, the order mandated enterprises, both private and public, to pay workers full wages. Factories, shopkeepers, owners of small and medium enterprises were asked not to cut any wages for the period of the lockdown;

landlords were asked to waive rents. At the same time, however, states were commanded by the central government to disallow any movement of people across border lines.

The afterthought – a critical delay of 120 hours – was too late to stem what would be the single largest mass exodus of people since the Partition of India in 1947. The sheer unenforceability of the fiat on compulsory wages made it meaningless. Save the exceptionalism of a benevolent employer – the 'seth' – as the workers called him, payments were frozen on the very day the lockdown started.

On the flip side, the bureaucratic ban on the movement of the poor only weaponized the police force against the most vulnerable and impoverished citizens, at the toughest moments of their already difficult lives. In any case, by the time the contradictory twin orders came it was already too late: the exodus was unstoppable.

The police restrictions made the Indian state an obstructionist micromanager – hostile, to be feared, and at times brutal. And the policy invisibilization of the poorest Indian citizen, paradoxically, made the same state absent where it should have been generous, present, available and accessible. This unwitting schizophrenia had lethal consequences and marked the beginning of a humanitarian crisis so big that it overshadowed the threat of COVID.

The morning after the prime minister's televised address to the nation, I drove out to the capital's borders. Delhi shares its boundary with Haryana on three edges and with Uttar Pradesh, the country's most populated state, on its eastern frontier. And there, where it should have had an overarching presence, officialdom had gone entirely missing. In the interiors of the city there were police at every street corner. In fact, through the pandemic, arbitrarily placed police barricades slowed down the movement of ambulances and cars rushing desperate patients to hospital or back. But at the borders of India's capital, for the first forty-eight hours at least, there were no men or women in khaki. Nor were there any helpdesks, doctors, aid workers or local administrators who might have been able to point out night shelters or sources of drinking water to the migrants on the road. No one thought to convert petrol pumps into temporary rest houses, or to allow the roadside dhabas all along India's highways to remain open so that there was at least basic mainstay food available on the long march home for the migrants.

Instead, it was a maelstrom of despair, anguish and anger.

For as far as the eye could see, people were walking, tiny and diminished against the giant backdrop of the flyovers they left behind.

In the beginning there was not even the cursory border checkpost. Just desolation on the highways, broken every few metres by the sight of people leaving, marching under bridges, jumping over steep ledges and open drains, their rage alternating only with their helplessness.

India was possibly the only country in the world to shutter public transport during this time. Thirteen thousand five hundred passenger trains of the railways suddenly stopped running. Mumbai's local trains, which ferry 7.5 million passengers every day, were now inoperational. Bengaluru's 6,000 buses that cater to 5 million citizens daily went off the roads. And the capital's metro services, which enable the mobility of 5.7 million Delhiites daily, were halted. City planners pointed out that to maintain a one-metre separation between individuals, a globally templated norm of 'social distancing', Mumbai's suburban trains would need to increase capacity by roughly sixteen times and Bengaluru's bus fleet by four times.

Not all of those who left for home immediately upon announcement of the lockdown knew that there would be no inter-state buses, trains or flights. At the Veer Hakikat Bus Terminal in Delhi, families huddled together on the pavement as the natural light dimmed. The women hid their faces behind ghunghats while the men sat on their haunches, their arms outstretched. Their children squatted beside them on the road, their pocket-sized bodies the same height as the small cloth sacks that had been packed for the journey. '*Aap maharaj log hai, aap hamein ghar pahuncha sakte hain,*' (You are like kings and queens compared to us, you can help us reach our homes) one of them pleaded.

On Instagram, celebrities baked banana bread in their version of the ordinary. Upper middle class, startled by how the skies had cleared of smog the moment vehicles were off the roads, added 'Covid Blue' to their list of rainbow cheer. Netflix was now an adverb, like Google.

Out on India's highways, from the north to the south, in a parallel universe, millions of Indians had begun the long march for both survival and solace.

Most surged right ahead, walking so fast I was out of breath trying to keep pace.

'Have you ever known a politician or his son to die during a calamity?' twenty-six-year-old Rajneesh Rajput Singh, a worker in the Maruti Suzuki automobile factory, snarled at me, as I panted between sentences, trying to keep up with him. Singh was a man in a hurry; the walk to his village in Bareilly, Uttar Pradesh, would take four days. It was nearly 300 kilometres away. He had no time for niceties. 'Each one of them, these politicians, should be made to serve in the military. Send them to the borders in Ladakh. Let them understand what hardship is.

Maybe then they would treat us better. If the government could not, why weren't our companies asked to arrange buses to take us home? Are we being made to walk like this just because we are poor? Are we being humiliated because we are poor? Are we being sent to die because we are poor?'

In that instant, it was clear that one was bearing witness to the beginnings of a catastrophe. The medical crisis of COVID seemed to pale in contrast. Panicked and helpless, but also acutely mindful of my own privilege, I took pictures and furiously tweeted the chief ministers of Delhi and its neighbouring states. There was no response.

'Poverty will kill me now, the virus will take time,' said Rajneesh, seething with cynicism. In the next three months, I would hear that sentiment over and over again, whether in the slums of Dharavi, the graveyards of Hyderabad, the forests of Bhiwandi or the factories of Telangana. Whether it was the textile worker in Surat or the science graduate in Mumbai, the perspective was the same. COVID was less lethal than economic deprivation and social displacement. In the eight months between March and October 2020, cumulative household incomes in India dropped by approximately 22 per cent. And for those among the poorest 10 per cent, per capita incomes dropped by 42 per cent, nearly halving.[8]

'Walking in this heat for four days is almost certain to take my life,' Rajneesh said. 'But what option do I have?' Rajneesh didn't know it then, but as hundreds of thousands of Indians began to leave the cities, one feeble, ill-planned attempt was made to organize buses to transport the workers to their villages. But instead of basic common-sense measures ensuring single-file lines and allowing the movement of only a few hundred at a time, and barricades and yellow ribbons every kilometre and use of the military and paramilitary for crowd control, policemen with sticks and loudspeakers stood by languidly as the throng of humanity pressed ahead. The barren highway leading up to the capital's Anand Vihar bus stop was hit by a deluge. As word got out that buses may be available in the capital, it wasn't just the local migrant workers, thousands of men and women, many of whom had already walked a couple of hundred kilometres from states further north, descended on the terminal in East Delhi. Desperate people pressed and pushed ahead, falling on top of each other, in a near stampede. In cities like Mumbai, similar scenes of chaos erupted at railway stations, with workers demanding a passage home.

And then the State gave up.

Worse, the poor, invisible to policy planners in the first week of the lockdown, were now judged and tarnished by elite commentators, who insinuated that they were virus carriers because they had congregated in such large numbers. Orphaned by the state to begin with, they were now being vilified.

As the floodgates burst open to release an explosion of millions of people on the highways of the country, the government fell back on its earlier approach – to police them into staying back.

It failed spectacularly.

Fundamental economic security may have been the trigger for exodus. No one paused to consider that in a life-and-death crisis, everyone wanted to be home with their loved ones. The unsaid assumption by policymakers was that this sentiment was a privilege of only the middle class and wealthy.

Luckily for Ranveer Singh, he'd already managed to make it to Agra. He was just 80 kilometres short of home and thought he'd catch a night's sleep at the railway station. Pinki and Mamata shared the news with the family as sister and wife thought about what they'd prepare for lunch to welcome him home.

They may not have had more than a few hundred rupees in savings, or much more than a pack of biscuits or bread to see them through, but India's impoverished citizens were determined to do what it took to get home. Whether they had to beg, borrow, bribe or be beaten up, they walked.

And the lockdown shifted from being a welfare measure intended to prepare the public health system for a pandemic to becoming a coercive and punitive display of official apathy – and, in some cases, brutality.

Already pushed into penury, the poor now had to contend with hostile, aggressive policemen.

Outside Delhi's Lok Nayak Hospital, so named after Jayprakash Narayan, the socialist 'people's leader' from the 1970s, I met a man squatting on the road and leaning against the police barricade placed at the entrance gate. He was weeping inconsolably. His mask was now slung around his neck and his eyes were brimming with tears. Wearing trousers rolled up to the knees, he kept leaning forward to touch a bandage wrapped around one of them. His name was Manoj and he was the driver of an electric rickshaw with a home in the byzantine, crowded quarters of Old Delhi. With the lockdown in place, it had been many days since Manoj had been able to earn even a paisa. That morning when he left the house, it was not to make a trip to the hospital. Manoj decided to walk a few extra kilometres to a wholesale vegetable market in the hope that the prices of basic essentials would be cheaper there than at the retail outlets in his neighbourhood. Manoj wept like a child. 'They thrashed me, they took their lathis and beat me and bruised me. I was only trying to find a way to feed my family.'

The police turned their baton on Manoj for violating the lockdown. Then they pushed him into a rickshaw and left him at the gate of the hospital so he could be treated for the injuries they had inflicted on him.

Manoj pointed to the gashes and bruises on his leg and to his inflamed, swollen wrist, clearly red from the violence. The hospital was now a full COVID facility, turning away all patients other than those who were infected by the virus. Because the police had brought him in, the doctors gave him first aid and then shooed him away. The security staff nudged him out of the gate and asked him to go to a non-COVID hospital to get help. Manoj thought the police might have broken a bone or torn a ligament. 'I'm in acute pain. I have four small children, what will I do, where will I go, how will I feed them?'

There was no way for Manoj to get to a different hospital to get an X-ray done. With his knee hurt, he couldn't walk. And in any case, he feared he might be thrashed at the next police barricade too. He hobbled home and rubbed some limestone on his wounds.

Human rights groups documented at least twenty deaths across the country that took place during the seventy-day lockdown.[9] Seventeen of these were from beating or caning by the police on the streets; three happened in police custody.

Missing at the borders through the first crucial week, men in khaki now took position as gatekeepers to keep the 'barbarians' behind the metaphorical city gates. Rampukar Yadav, a construction worker from Begusarai in Bihar, was among those walking the 1,200 kilometres home when he received a phone call from his wife. He had left the city without any money and had packed some dry chapatis with salt to see him through the journey. The news got worse: their boy, one-year-old Rampavesh, was critically ill. Yadav collapsed in grief, begging the cops to let him past the barricade. But they shoved him back, beat him and dismissed him with a '*Chal hat, maderchod*, do you think you are a VIP that we should let you through'. His child died before he could get back.

Mann Kumari, pregnant with her fourth baby, left Ambala in Haryana for her home in Madhya Pradesh with her husband Sanjay and three small children, on foot. She had walked close to 150 kilometres when her water broke. They were on the highway, near Aligarh in Uttar Pradesh, with no hospital, doctor or shelter in sight. She had no choice but to deliver right there on the side of the tarred road with the help of a few other women who were walking in the same cluster as she was.

Sitting with her children by the wayside, a polyester print sari tied around her slender frame, she broke down, wondering how to organize food for her small children. She held her newest-born, Shivam, to her breast, to feed him. But where would she get milk for the other three, she asked me. The children, three boys, had spent the night on the pavement, sleeping on a sack, leaning against the support of downed shop shutters, finding a tiny space for themselves between cycles and metallic odds and ends there. Except for the newborn, who was wrapped in a soft blue towel, the children were bare-chested. Was she able to rest at all, we asked, after giving birth? Mann Kumari smiled sadly. 'Not even for a few hours.'

Between the five family members – now six with the birth of their boy – they had a single bicycle. Sanjay was a brick-kiln worker in Haryana, who, unlike so many others, did not leave immediately and waited to see if things might get better. When they did not, he stuffed their belongings into little cloth bags – biscuits, a handful of clothes, some kerosene, a cooking utensil and ladle – and tied them with thick rope to the handle and spokes of his cycle. More than a mode of transport the cycle was something like a suitcase on wheels. He would push the cycle as the family walked.

Mann Kumari pulled out a cauldron from a jute bag tied to the handlebar of the cycle. They had a little rice left. She began preparing that day's meal. There were still 800 kilometres left to walk.

And there was Jyoti Paswan, the teenager who made her father, Mohan Paswan, sit on the back of a bicycle, strung a basket of essentials to the front and rode 1,200 kilometres from Delhi to her village in Darbhanga in Bihar. Mohan, a rickshaw driver, had just recovered from a knee surgery and was unable to either walk or ride the cycle himself. It took eight harrowing days, crippling both mentally and physically for a fifteen-year-old schoolgirl. She did the marathon in rubber slippers, wearing the same set of clothes – a pair of cotton trousers, a T-shirt and a scarf wrapped over it – for the entire week. But, perhaps a collective need to avoid feelings of guilt made the nation cast her saga as a story of triumph instead of tragedy. She even got the attention of Ivanka Trump, the somewhat vapid, entitled daughter of Donald Trump, who tweeted about Jyoti as if she were the new wonder woman from *Avengers* instead of a traumatized survivor. '*Kya karte?*' Jyoti asked me, once safely back home. 'Everything hurt – my feet, my hands – but how many days could we have waited in the hope that buses or trains would start?' They would sleep at petrol pumps every night and depend on passers-by for something as basic as a glass of water. 'I kept my strength by looking at everyone else who was walking on the highways,' she said, looking down with a shy smile, still in the days before she became a cause celebre and the subject of proposed Bollywood flicks. 'I cried often. But what choice did I have?'

There were so many others whose stories never got told, reduced to mere statistics, tally marks in their own tragic tales, unseen and unheard. Under the shadow of skyscrapers and apartment buildings with names like Magnolia, Laburnum and Camellia, they walked in pursuit of exactly what the wealthy seek during a crisis – dignity, security, family.

On the national highway linking the capital to the automobile hub of Gurugram, where luxury SUVs and shiny sedans are rolled out in the thousands every year, I met Seema, her husband Premvir and their four small children as they took cover under the shade of a tree, pausing in the summer heat to take a sip of water from a leaky municipal pipe. Seema filled an empty two-litre plastic bottle of coke with the slightly muddy water, held her four-year-old close to her, pulled the pallu of her sari over her eyes to block the heat and hobbled ahead. 'My feet are hurting,' said their ten-year-old son Kamal, collapsing in the next few metres on the pavement. Before the pandemic shut down his work, Prem, a worker from Bareilly in Uttar Pradesh, worked as a scrap seller in the city, collecting used newspapers and bottles and recycling them for a small fee. Instead of crossing the border, first into Delhi and then into their home state, they were heading back to their one-room accomodation, where they'd have to beg the landlord to let them stay on without rent and where there would be no food to give the children. This was the third time the police had turned them away from the border. As a mother, Seema was despairing. 'They abused us, waved their lathis at us, shooed us away and told us they'd thrash us if we didn't leave,' she said, sobbing into her cotton sari. 'How will I look after my children?' Faced with the rawness of her grief, the norms of distancing seemed like an elite and sanitized concept. I placed a hesitant arm around her and she cried like a child. Her teenage daughter, with a vacant stare in her eyes, pointed to the blisters on her small feet. '*Chalte chalte thak gaye.*' (We are so tired from all the walking.)

On 31 March, Solicitor General Tushar Mehta told the Supreme Court that there were 'no migrants on the road, as of 11 a.m. that morning'.

This was absolutely untrue.

Across thirteen states, travelling 30,000 kilometres, we were witness to how the country's highways became veritable refugee camps for the displaced masses. Near Udaipur, cement workers chased a truck down the expressway, desperate for a seat, willing to offer literally anything in exchange and falling back crestfallen when declined by the driver for fear of police reprisal. In Bhiwandi, I met women carrying giant steel trunks on their heads as they marched through the darkness of forestland, walking at night to avoid the scorching sun in the day. In Telangana, workers who were going home with just two white plastic buckets, uncovered them to show me what they were travelling back with: a blanket, a shovel and a spade. 'We are ready to work to earn a living. But no one is willing to let us work.' In a factory in Delhi, an infrastructure giant locked his workers behind a giant steel wall so that they could not step out and try and make their way home. When we made our way inside the compound to tell their story we too were locked in with them and our cameras snatched away.

For the thirty-seven days that all public transport between the states of India remained shut – and even for several weeks after that – the scenes on the country's highways were a blot on our collective conscience.

Across India, workers sold their phones, the only possession they had that was of some monetary value. Some bartered them for food, others for places on private trucks that smuggled them out like trafficked children, one on top of the other.

And on 8 May, nearly two months after the claim by India's senior-most law officer that there were no workers walking the roads, a single frame said it all.

It was the sight of a stale chapati lying on a rail track in Aurangabad, yesterday's dinner packed as today's lunch by twenty men who were headed back home on foot from Maharashtra to their village in Madhya Pradesh. They had walked 45 kilometres; there was another 100 kilometres to cover before they would have been able to try their luck at getting a seat on a train. Instead of that, it was their corpses that were found on the tracks. Next to the scattered pieces of rotis, was a bottle of hair oil and a single slipper. These remains of the day were the belongings of tribal migrant workers from a remote Adivasi village. They had gone to sleep on the railway line at four in the morning, exhausted from all the walking. This was also a place where they thought they would not be noticed or disturbed by the police. A goods train ran over them an hour later.

It was a haunting tragedy.

Who were these men? Where did they come from? What were their names? What must their families be going through?

Shahdol district in Madhya Pradesh is a mineral-rich region in central India. It is flush with coal, fire clay, ochre and marble. Nearly half of its population is tribal. One of the Adivasi villages in this remote corner of the Deccan plateau is Antoli, where only 193 families live; 75 per cent of its population belongs to the Gond tribe.

It was eighteen hours from Delhi by road over potholes, through puddles and past flyovers that appeared to be under a permanent state of incomplete construction before the path opened up to the breathtakingly unspoilt Kaimur mountains of the Vindhya range. The length and roughness of the journey were daunting. We thought of turning back and terminating it more than once. Even from the last motorable point we had to walk another few hours on foot before we reached Antoli. We made our way past small clusters of thorny thatched homes, children playing in the open fields, and over little rocky rivulets before arriving at the tiny hamlet of huts in the middle of vistas of wide-open green for miles beyond.

This is one of India's forgotten villages.

Among those who worked in the village and had not left for the city, more than 66 per cent were involved in marginal activity that provided livelihood for less than six months of the year.

The women gathered around the village well. Some held their infants in their laps, others allowed their children to scamper about. Nearly all of them had lost someone that night, when the velocity of the train crushed the men to death.

Chandravati sat on the edge of the well's parapet, crying into her orange-indigo sari. She wasn't precisely sure of her husband Deepak's age. Maybe he was twenty, or maybe he was twenty-five, no older. She herself was twenty-four. 'The country may have moved on. But I cannot forget this for as long as I live,' she said, a steely strength suddenly displacing the deep sorrow.

Rohit, a one-year-old wrapped in a white muslin cloth, looked around in wonderment and smiled. He did not yet know that his father Vijay would never be back home.

An old man sat on his haunches in the wet mud, a stick in hand. Everyone called him 'Chacha'. His two sons were among those who had died under the wheels of the train. He held his head and wept. Each family had been given ₹1,200,000 as compensation. It was the sort of money they could never have dreamt of when their boys were alive. 'What will I do with the money they have given as compensation? Bring my children back,' Chacha said, resting his head on his knees. 'Couldn't the two states have spoken and organized a way to send our children home by train?'

The trains that couldn't take them back while they were still alive were requisitioned to take their corpses from Aurangabad to Jabalpur, from where they were sent home to Shahdol and Umaria.

Trains became a poignant symbol of both tragedy and hope. Of what could have been. And what was.

On the same morning that Aurangabad woke up to news of the train running over sleeping workers from Antoli, in Gujarat – the prime minister's and home minister's home state – the state's first 'Shramik' train was leaving the station from Surat.

After weeks of chronicling migrant workers' long march home, as I stood on the platform and watched that first train to Bihar slowly pull away. I was overwhelmed. Tears streamed down my face – in relief, but also perhaps in a release of the gigantic sorrow I had witnessed.

Through the barricaded windows I spoke to the workers as the carriage inched forward. They were mostly millworkers, who had tried to leave on foot and then by bus, but had been held back by the police. Among them was a fourteen-year-old boy, Arun Kumar. Poverty had compelled him to come and find work in the city along with the adults from his village. Surely, you must have had a different dream for yourself, I asked, upset to see a child having to experience any of this, including needing to come to the city at all. 'I have just one dream – to get home.'

This is how the exodus during the lockdown shrank dreams, reducing them to aspirations of survival and security.

The government said the railways would subsidize 85 per cent of the cost of sending a worker home while the state governments would fund the remaining amount. In other words, the migrant workers, already in penury, without wages or food, were not expected to pay for their passage.

But that is not what happened.

At the Kalaburagi station in Karnataka I boarded a Shramik train headed to Lucknow in Uttar Pradesh. I had been granted a few minutes by the stationmaster to meet with people before the train left the platform. I was excited to walk through a crowded compartment, again in the hope that the trauma for these men, women and children would finally end. Some of them were toilet cleaners, others had been working as labour on a pipeline project. And then I spotted the ticket they clutched in their hands. The cost of the ticket was printed on it: ₹770. Officials had already explained to us that anyone could pay for the ticket – the Centre, the state, the worker, the worker's employer – but the ticket had to be accounted for. A quick show of hands revealed that the workers in the coach had all purchased their own tickets. Only a handful of men and women told us that the local legislator or their 'seth' had loaned or given them the money to buy their tickets. The majority of workers at this station, and every other I reported from, had taken a loan or had sold their mobile phones – the only asset they still owned – to raise money for the journey back. It was clear: despite the claims by politicians, migrant workers were being made to pay their way home. 'Of course we feel terrible; we have been through such hardship. I think it's obvious how much anyone cares for us,' said Wasiq, one of the workers headed home to Uttar Pradesh.

The tragedies did not end with the resuming of the train services.

Horror stories of heat and hunger emerged from the Shramik trains.

Qazi Anwar, forty-five, a construction worker from Mumbai, died on the train to Bihar. His friend Tauhir, who was among the ten people travelling with Anwar, said that what was meant to be a thirty-hour journey went on for four days. 'Anwar had a glass of sattu for ten rupees and boarded the train. After that there was no food available for us. We did not even get a glass of water.'

Tauhir said it was only when the train pulled up at stations that little children would run up and bring them water in plastic buckets. Anwar, he said, had died on Eid.

'Instead of Eid ki namaz, we have brought a body home.'

The most devastating image from that time was that of a baby trying to wake up his dead mother at a station platform in Bihar. Arbina Khatoon lay comatose as her child tugged at her. The railways said she had died from a heart attack, denying that the ordeal and trauma of the journey had killed her. Arbina's mother Shahrun told me it was exhaustion, heat and hunger that had taken away her daughter.

And then came the second major horrific accident, this time in Uttar Pradesh. 'We were treated worse than *lawaris janwar*,' Vikas Kalindi from Jharkhand, one of the few survivors from that incident, said. Twenty-six of his co-workers died when the trucks on which they had managed to purchase a passage home from Rajasthan overturned en route in Auraiya in Uttar Pradesh. No ambulances or paramedics were provided to pull the bodies out from the debris. Instead, the workers who had managed to make it out alive were asked to lift the mangled bodies. The dead were then bundled into plastic bags and thrown on slabs of ice at the back of another truck. Vikas was asked to sit there with the bodies. 'The stench overwhelmed me. I did not want to live. Are we not human beings too?'

From the railway station in Agra, Ranveer Singh felt a growing restlessness rise within him as he wrestled with some of the same questions. He called his sister again. 'Can you come and get me, come if you can, I don't feel so well suddenly.' He did not have the energy to walk further. Eighty kilometres meant a road trip of just over an hour, but given the curfew the family would need special permission from the district magistrate's office to organize the paperwork that would allow them past police barricades.

By the time their application moved, Ranveer had died. Right there at the railway station. The police said he'd had a heart attack.

Pinki is still haunted by his last words – 'Come and get me if you can;' haunted that she could not, did not; haunted at the thought of her brother's desperate loneliness in the minutes before his death; and haunted that all that remains of him today is his password-locked phone.

It needed his fingerprint to unlock.

On 14 September 2020, the government informed Parliament that it has no data on migrant deaths.

Two hundred and nine migrants died while walking back home; 97 died on the trains that were belatedly organized.[10]

And these cases are only the ones we know of.

In November 2020, when India was lulled into believing that the worst of the pandemic was in the past and when the ferociousness of the Delta variant had not yet hit home, Darbhanga, famous for its trade in fish, mangoes and makhana, but also for Jyoti Paswan, now officially the subject of a Bollywood biopic, got itself an airport. Within days of its inauguration, 30,000 people had flown through the terminal, with its single-storeyed building, once used only by the Indian Air Force.

Exactly a year after the teenager had cycled more than a thousand kilometres home, in March 2021, I went to meet Jyoti and her father in their village.

Unknown to us, we were just a few days away from the cascading surge of the second wave.

As we touched down on the air force-controlled runway, the irony was staggering. Exactly a year ago, even the bicycle that Jyoti rode was more than what millions of other workers had access to. Now there was a commercial liner on the tarmac.

We drove past lush green fields of wheat and leafy banana trees. In small government-run primary schools, the tinkle of children laughing had returned to the classroom. They didn't know then that it was a joy that would be short-lived. We sat peaceably at a railway line, where children sold guavas with black salt, and peanuts packed in scraps of paper and waited for the train to whistle past us. Again, my mind harked back to the time when the tracks had become a virtual metaphor for tragedy.

We were driving to the village of Sirhulli, and on the highway we saw girls on their bicycles making their way to school, their dupattas tied in a knot to the side of their neatly pressed kurtas so as to not get entangled in the spokes. These were like dreams on wheels, a far cry from the trauma that Jyoti had been forced to endure. The programme to distribute free bicycles in Bihar had increased the probability of a girl enrolling for secondary education and actually staying till the end of that grade by 32 per cent.

At the entrance to their village, Jyoti, dressed in a white shirt and black trackbottoms, was cycling in small circles around the block, waiting for us to arrive. Most of the hutments were made from straw and mud. The Paswan house, still under construction, stood out for being the only concrete building in the locality, its freshly assembled bricks towering above the others.

'I am happy today,' said Jyoti as we sat side by side, leaning against the hand pump in a small courtyard. A few stained plastic buckets lay tossed right next to it. In another corner of the compound, a wailing infant was being given an oil massage.

'I was so scared last year about everything – food and water and how we would survive. 'Now we have what we need,' she said, smiling and looking around at the modest surroundings, the clothes drying on the brambles behind us, and at the damp, dark stairway leading to a tiny kitchen and a large mattress on the floor. The global media attention her ordeal fetched meant that offers of help poured in, along with more bicycles than she would ever need or have space to keep.

For Jyoti, there is always a shadow hanging over the possibilities of the future. Scratch the surface and the horrors of the previous year are never too far behind. 'I am a girl. Anyone could have done anything to me along the way, anything they wanted,' she said softly, 'even my father was really scared.'

Jyoti's mother will never forget her struggle to feed their five children during that time. Phoolo wore yellow lacquer bangles on her wrist and a red bindi on her forehead. She busied herself in the kitchen, making us milky tea and samosas. Flour and pulses were stored in plastic bags hung from hooks created from nails in the open brick wall. A pink bicycle was parked on its stand among the vessels and plates. 'We lived in abject poverty,' she said, recounting how the family worked as labour in the wheat and paddy fields and carried mud and cement at construction sites to earn a few rupees a day. It was this penury that had compelled Mohan to leave for the city.

Mohan had tried his hand at a host of odd jobs. He was a factory worker in the Maruti automobile factory. His smile travelled up to his eyes as he remembered the months he worked as a chef in an Italian restaurant. 'I could make pasta and pizza,' he told us with a broad grin. Finally, he settled on driving an electric rickshaw. And then he had a terrible accident. He pulled his pants up to his knee to show us the post-surgery stitches. After the accident and the operation, he could no longer function as a driver because bending his knee was impossible. He was planning to return to the village, when the lockdown was imposed.

Economic hardship does not tell the complete story of India's impoverished classes. A survey of 8,000 migrant workers revealed that a vast majority – 81 per cent – who fled the cities for their villages at the peak of the lockdown were from marginalized caste groups, scheduled castes, scheduled tribes or other backward castes (OBCs).[11]

Mohan Paswan, a Dalit, saw shades of his own life in those statistics. 'There was a time that *bade log* kept their distance from us; we were not considered clean or pure enough,' he said matter-of-factly and without rancour. 'We did not experience this in the city. But here in the village, my family has been discriminated against. It's a lot less than before. And after Jyoti has become famous, people are really nice to us.'

Jyoti, who had just cleared her class ten exams in such excruciating circumstances, was keen to show us her school. This time she hopped on to a scooter and we followed. It was a single white building with arched corridors and a big lawn – this is where she was happiest, she told us. 'I just want to study. I hope all girls are able to study.'

That evening, before we left Darbhanga, Jyoti Yadav and I went for a cycle ride, she on her favourite blue one, I on a red one borrowed from the assortment of options she now owns. I was mindful of not romanticizing her life and of inadvertently channelling her resilience into some sort of redemption for the state, or for any of us. Yet, as we felt the wind in our hair, for a few brief moments it felt like something that was approximate to freedom and hope.

But at the home of Mukesh Mandal, the migrant worker who had died by suicide 365 days ago, there were no signs of freedom or hope. Saraswati Kunj seemed frozen in time, with the same open sewer and garbage landfills marking the entrance to Mandal's home. This time, Poonam, his widow, took me inside the room adjacent to where she and her children sleep; the room where he had spent his last moments alive. A small pink ceiling fan whirred from the bamboo pole as sunlight crept in through the gaps in the thatched roof. It's the pole that Mukesh had used to take his life. Inside, where she and her four children shared a single room with her parents, a half-eaten slice of papaya infested with flies sat on the window ledge. From a blue chipped wall hung a plastic bag which held some raw peas. Outside, her littlest one desperately lunged at a small circular steel tiffin to grab small bites of roti and vegetables. Did they have enough to have two meals a day, I asked Poonam. 'Not always,' she said, staring at her toes, as we sat on the the doorframe ledge. Another toddler rolled in the mud next to us. Poonam had attempted to work as a domestic help, cook, cleaner and sweeper in the high-rise mansions that formed the outer periphery of where she lived. But those attempts have gone nowhere because she still did not have an Aadhaar card, the government-recognized biometric identity card that nearly all prospective employers insisted on.

Sometimes she could not get past the imposing carved gates that opened up to palm trees, boulevards, gymnasiums and pools. Security guards scanned cars and watched every entrant hawk-like. She had no identification that was considered legitimate.

Her family was not the only one trapped under the economic debris of the first wave. Seventy-five per cent of workers surveyed in March 2021 said they had no access to a steady source of income; 31 per cent said they had no access to healthcare.[12]

Sunita, Poonam's mother, was keen that the family go back to their village in Bihar. Her husband, Poonam's father, she told us, is now an alcoholic. *'Mera boodha daru pee kar para rehta hai.'* (My doddering old husband just drinks through his days.) Poonam's father spent his days begging for alms at the local temple, bringing back a few rupees on a good day for the kids. Poonam had been abandoned by her husband's family, who blame her for Mukesh Mandal's suicide. Sunita tried to supplement the household income by pulling a cart of vegetables on a cycle with Pinky, another single mother to two children. The only time Poonam smiled is when her children pulled out a picture album and shared their memories of old, happier moments with their father.

It was just a few days later that state-wise restrictions began to be announced as the contours of the second wave of the pandemic started to take ominous shape. This time the government, singed by the burns of its mistakes in 2020, did not opt for a countrywide lockdown. States were given the option to localize restrictions on movement and commerce as they thought appropriate. Nor was public transport closed.

In cities across India, workers, who had barely returned to the cities from their villages, started to queue up again outside bus terminals and railway stations. Why were they leaving this time, I asked, when there was no lockdown in place?

'Hamara vishwas toot gaya hai,' they said. 'Our trust has been broken.'

At the time of writing this book, COVID had ravaged India for over two years, peaking in the months between March and June in both 2020 and 2021. The soldiers of India's battle against the virus were a phalanx of healthcare workers – community activists, nurses, doctors, ward boys, ambulance drivers and security staff. But despite accolades pouring in for them right from the top – the prime minister famously urged the country to light a diya or bang a thali in solidarity with healthcare personnel on 5 April 2020 – on the ground, medical personnel had to face relentless stigma and violence. In the early months of the pandemic there was so much prejudice and ignorance that doctors and nurses who died from COVID were sometimes denied a dignified cremation or burial. Many came home in disguise from hospital duty. Scientists repeatedly warned that a high number of infections would almost invariably mean that the virus would mutate. And in the first quarter of 2021, B.1.617.2, or the Delta variant, hit India like a storm. If hospital beds were the main shortage during the first wave, in the Delta surge everything ran out – from oxygen to drugs – leaving front-line workers exposed once again to the wrath and despair of patients. Citizens experienced the second wave as a sharp, intense burst of violence because of the compressed time and space it unfolded in. But from the point of view of health workers, the number of lives lost among them in the line of duty was nearly equal in both waves. By the end of 2021, the Indian Medical Association said 1,700 doctors in the country had died from COVID. Exhausted health workers began preparing for a third wave, this time by the highly transmissible but likely milder variant called Omicron. As the new wave swirled around India's hospitals, ominously threatening a high tide, resident doctors were forced to protest on the streets, sometimes clashing with policemen, against massive shortages in the workforce.

3

The First Responders

On the sixth floor of Cama Hospital in Mumbai, the elevator still bears the scars of the wounds that Ajmal Kasab's AK-47 inflicted on it when he turned his automatic rifle on the door and shot right through it on the night of 26 November 2008. It's taken Yogita Bagad, who was twenty-three years old when the city came under siege from Pakistani terrorists, more than a decade to be able to enter the hospital without noticing the gaping holes in the lift.

It was 9.30 at night, Yogita had just stepped out of the ward to grab a quick bite when the watchman came running up the steps, panting in panic. A man with a gun had shot two security guards; they all needed to hide. There were thirty-five young mothers and their newborns in Yogita's ward. It was just she and another staff nurse on night duty. Yogita had no notion of what a terrorist was, apart from what she'd vaguely seen and heard from time to time on the news. But her survival instincts kicked in. She herded all the mothers and babies out of their beds into a tiny, unventilated storage room at the end of the corridor and flicked the lights off.

Outside, the cracks of gunfire filled the empty hospital corridors. Periodically, they could hear men screaming and pounding on closed doors. Yogita gathered the mobile phones of the women and quickly motioned for them to switch them to the silent mode. But there was still a problem: the infants were barely a few days old; what if one of them burst out crying and brought attention to where they were crouched in complete darkness? By now Yogita knew which of the mothers were lactating. If the babies were being breastfed, they'd be quiet.

It was because of this quick thinking that they all survived that fateful November night, when ten Pakistani terrorists stepped off a dinghy at the Gateway of India, in a meticulously planned act of war against India.

As the police, close on his heels, took aim at Kasab to stop him, he hurled hand grenades down the hospital floor and the entire building started shaking from the impact of their explosion. Yogita had managed a quick call to her mother to say her goodbye. 'I don't think I will make it back alive tonight,' she whispered hurriedly into the phone, through tears. Her mother sobbed at the other end.

It was past 2 a.m. when the commandos let them all out from their closet-sized hiding space into safety.

Yogita believed this brush with death prepared her for anything life would throw at her. Twelve years later, still working with new mothers and babies, she is much more terrified of what she calls the 'battle that does not seem to end.'

It took Yogita six months and several sessions with the hospital therapist to 'come out' from the trauma of the 26/11 terror attack. 'That period I could leave behind. But with COVID-19, *yeh lagta hai kabhi khatam nahin hoga.* (It feels like this will never end.) Every day, when I leave the hospital, I worry about having picked up an infection that I will take home to my mother. It's like living with constant fear.'

One-thousand six-hundred kilometres away in the south, in the city of Chennai, Dr Pradeep Kumar was also grappling with a fear he had never known. As a surgeon he had seen death more times than he could count; but this was a paralysing, heart-stopping jolt to his very being.

Pradeep and his best friend, Dr Simon Hercules, worked at the super-speciality Brain and Spine Centre of New Hope Hospital in Chennai's Kilpauk area, not far from the serene Chetpet lake and the Votive Shrine. This church was built as an offering to Mother Mary at another point in history when Chennai, then known as Madras, was debilitated by apprehension of what lay ahead. The Japanese had just entered the Second World War and their fleet was sailing towards Trincomalee, the coastal peninsular town of Tamilian settlers, now in Sri Lanka. The church's archbishop records how 'Madras was in the grip of a scare. Schools with their boarders were evacuated into the interior. The exodus of people was such that Madras looked for a while like a depopulated city.'

This was December 1942.

But what happened during the war was nothing compared with the paranoia, suspicion and fright that took over Chennai in the year of the pandemic.

Simon, fifty-five, was a God-fearing, church-going all-round nice guy with the reputation of never saying no to patients. At the height of the lockdown, when elective surgeries had been stopped across hospitals in India, Simon would ring Pradeep, an orthopaedic surgeon, and cajole him to turn up for operations. When all else failed, Simon would fall back on emotional pressure. 'He is my relative, he is known to me, I need your help,' he would say, urging Pradeep and other hesitant colleagues to get to the hospital. Through the early days of the pandemic, when private medical facilities effectively stopped treating anyone but COVID patients, Simon never turned anyone away and never put his operations on pause. In fact, he picked up the infection from a patient who flew in from outside India for a surgery. As Simon's fever and cold got worse he was admitted to Apollo Hospital, an upscale private health chain where, after two weeks, on 19 April 2020, he lost the battle against the virus.

It was a Sunday when he died, the day Simon would normally have been at church. Pradeep, Simon's wife Anandi and their teenage son followed the ambulance to the Christian Cemetery in Kilpauk Garden Road, a sprawling sixteen-acre haven just behind the T.P. Chatram police station. The upscale grounds were fitted with surveillance cameras and high-speed internet to allow for families abroad to witness the last rites of their loved ones from thousands of miles away and in real time. But the trappings of modernity could not cloak the medieval coarseness of what happened next.

Just before he was placed on the ventilator, Simon had recorded a video message for Anandi. 'If I do not survive, please bury me according to the rituals of my faith,' he implored her. To fulfil his last wish, the local priest gave his consent for a spot in the burial ground to be set aside for Simon. But as they neared the grounds of the cemetery, a crowd of nearly a hundred men and women had gathered at the gates to stop the ambulance from entering. Steeped in ignorance about how COVID might spread, the local residents were on the rampage.

The health inspectors suggested diverting the ambulance to Velangadu cemetery, which was a ten-minute drive away in Anna Nagar. Night had fallen by now and the burial site was steeped in darkness. The mechanical diggers and excavators, colloquially known as JCBs (after Joseph Cyril Bamford, a British multinational manufacturer), got to work under Pradeep's supervision. WHO guidelines had stringent protocols for COVID burials; no bathing or embalming of the corpse was permitted and the grave had to be 12 feet deep, as opposed to the usual 6 feet. Only five people were allowed to be present and they had to be in personal protective equipment (PPE) from head to toe. The ambulance had been there less than fifteen minutes when they heard the sound of screaming in the distance. A mob of close to thirty men, armed with iron rods and sticks, were charging towards them. Before they could react, Pradeep, the ambulance driver Dhamu, Simon's wife and son, and the proclaimers working the gravedigging machines, all came under assault. Stones were hurled at them as the crowd raced towards them, caught hold of each of them and began to thrash them. Dhamu's head was bleeding from a gash, a ribbon of red now trailing down his neck. Pradeep gathered Simon's body in his arms, and the others helped him and they raced back to the vehicles. The healthcare workers who were deployed to ensure funeral protocols were attacked next. As the mob surrounded them and hit them with long wooden sticks, Pradeep and the others pushed their way past them, running on to the road, shouting in helpless despair at anyone prepared to listen. 'Help us, save, please save our lives.'

The ambulance was also battered; its windows were broken and its windshield smashed to bits. It was open to the elements from all sides. The hotline number 909 466, 7074 scrawled across the back in faded yellow, was the only thing that remained intact on its now broken frame.

At the back, Simon's body lay covered with sharp-edged

shrapnel of glass that stuck to the white plastic Ziplock his coffin had been wrapped in. The driver jumped on to the front seat and started the van, trying to ignore the blood splattered across the seat. The second ambulance driver also had a head injury. Pradeep followed in his own car, mindful that the drivers needed urgent first aid.

On their way out he worked the phone lines to the police and to state health ministry officials, who promised to send a battalion of uniformed men to the burial site. Pradeep dropped off the drivers at the hospital, jumped into the ambulance himself and drove with his foot on the accelerator. He had requested two ward boys who used to work with Simon to meet him at the hospital.

A rush of tears streams down Pradeep's face when he recounts what followed. With no manpower left and with no one else willing to take the risk, Pradeep zipped up in the PPE suit that had been kept aside for the gravedigger, took the wheel of the same pummelled ambulance, asked the ward staff to keep an eye on Simon's body, and drove back. They were going to make a third attempt to give their beloved friend the burial he had wanted.

This time the police had managed to clear the crowd. But Pradeep realized he was the only one in protective clothing. The JCB had been destroyed by the mob and its operators had fled from the grounds. No one was available to bury Simon. Pradeep was trembling. It was dark, the day was ending, and he could not leave Simon there. Choking on his tears, he knelt on the gravelly floor and started digging with his bare hands, completing the job the machines had begun. He had no shovels or spades. As he gathered mud with both hands and threw it over Simon's body to close the grave, he kept thinking the mob would come back for him. They could get reinforcements, return in larger numbers, maybe even force the police to flee. 'On the one hand I was so scared for my life. I was convinced they would come back and kill me,' he told me. 'But I just could not leave my friend there. If the police were not there, I know we would not have made it out alive.'

What shook Pradeep more than anything else was that Simon's son, not yet sixteen, had to see his father denied dignity in death. He had seen things he should never have seen at this age – the collective, coarse, violent ugliness of human beings, when panic turns to prejudice. In the rampaging crowd were women in their cotton nighties, holding sticks and charging towards fifty-year-old Anandi. Mother and son had to leave before they could say goodbye to Simon. 'As a doctor, death is not new to us. But fear, this fear, this fear is such a thing.'

Denied dignity in death and respect in life, doctors began to wonder if it might not be better for them to go unsung, unnoticed, unremarked on. After living through the hell of what happened to his friend, Pradeep folded both hands, and he looked broken as he bent over and said to me, 'I have a request for the media. When we die, can you all not mention it; if we can't be treated as human beings, it's best if we are allowed to go quietly.'

Pradeep's entreaty stood in cruel juxtaposition to the dramatic moment when tens of millions of Indians, urged by Prime Minister Modi, had stepped out on the balconies of their apartment buildings, the patios of their homes, the public parks of their neighbourhood and the walk-through narrow alleys of their slum tenements to light candles and bang thalis in salutation to healthcare workers at the front line of the country's fight against COVID. Whether it was a municipal sweeper who rolled a thin sliver of cotton into a tiny earthen lamp filled with a drop of kerosene and let its soft glow light up the ledge of her one-room shanty or Mukesh Ambani, the wealthiest man in India and the tenth richest in the world, who bowed before the gentle flicker of a candle, it seemed as if, in the symbolism of the moment, a country truly stood united – by fear, yes, but also by hope and gratitude.

But in truth, during the first wave, doctors, nurses and ward boys, claimed as heroes on paper, were treated as pariahs. In the summer of 2020, if health workers tested COVID positive, as many did, from standing at the first tier of defence against a marauding virus, they were treated like outcasts. In fact, India was perhaps the only country in the world where COVID birthed a new caste system, a new social order and a new kind of untouchability. Nurses who returned home from COVID duty, or worse, COVID recovery, were evicted from their rental homes. Some were asked not to enter the neighbourhood parks. Many lived in the shadow of the mob, fighting two adversaries at once – a recalcitrant virus and the contagion of bigotry.

In Delhi, we met a male nurse in the cloak of darkness on condition that we would not reveal his identity. In a middle-income neighbourhood in the north-east of the city, we stood and spoke under the dim light of a street lamp. Even with his mask on and face entirely covered, the nurse kept his back to our camera throughout our conversation. He met us at some distance from the apartment complex he lived in. Such was the viciousness of the stigma against health workers in the early months of COVID. A sputtering of blood in his cough compelled a COVID test. Now he was home, fully recovered, after fifteen days in hospital. 'I tried to keep positive by listening to music competition videos and hearing soothing music.' He had looked forward to sleeping in his own bed, grateful that he was back on his feet. But his neighbours had other plans. In his absence notices were plastered across the door of his home, ostensibly to inform everyone to keep their distance. In the meantime, a complaint was registered at the local police station. The neighbours started pressuring the landlord to evict the nurse from the premises. 'They look at me as if I am a thief, as if I am a petty criminal,' the nurse, originally from Kerala, but based in Delhi, said. 'I felt so awkward.' The nurse was able to stay on in his housing society because his landlord happened to be a doctor. The neighbours remained hostile. 'I am not angry,' he said, 'this is their ignorance.'

In Surat, Dr Sanjibani Panigrahi, posted at the city's Civil Hospital, was taunted and intimidated every day by men who would wait outside her building as she returned home from backbreaking hours at work. Finally, she tagged the prime minister on Twitter – Gujarat, after all, is his home state – compelling the local BJP legislator to step in and offer protection. Things calmed down for a bit. But then one evening, the neighbour who lived across the landing from her own apartment, accosted her as she climbed up the steps. As she rushed into her flat and locked the door behind her, he stood at her doorway and hurled expletives at her as his wife looked on mutely. Sanjibani pulled out her phone and started filming him, which set him off some more. He lunged at her, pushing her back as he tried to grab her phone, and shouted louder, '*Tu kya samajhti hai apne aap ko, tujhe yahan rehne nahin denge*,' (Who do you think you are? We won't let you stay here) he said. He was an unremarkable looking middle-aged man wearing a baby pink T-shirt neatly tucked into the waistband of trousers worn too high. 'We won't allow this. We know you must have COVID.' The man had been Sanjibani's neighbour for two years and they had always lived amicably, almost cheek by jowl. Sanjibani's three-year-old son started to cry at the sight of his mother being shouted at and jostled about. 'That hurt the most,' Sanjibani told me. 'I had to call the police. I was scared, I was disgusted, but I was determined.' She knew her child needed answers to make sense of what he had just witnessed. 'Uncle was very scared,' Sanjibani explained to her son. 'Sometimes when people get very scared, they become angry.'

'The pandemic has unleashed a collective fury in us,' Sanjibani said. 'I am unable to understand why this has happened. I understand there is fear. But there is fear all over the world. I haven't seen violence against doctors anywhere else. As a country we preach non-violence but we don't practise it. I just want to tell India, there is a war going on, but doctors are not your enemy.'

The highest number of COVID-related attacks on medical workers anywhere in the world took place in India. A quarter of all such assaults on health workers during the pandemic – 128 out of the 412 such recorded incidents in 2020 – gave India an ignominious top position on this global chart.[13]

In Indore, Dr Trupti Katdare and Dr Zakiya Sayed, best friends and colleagues, were on a field visit to Tatpatti Bhakal, a COVID hotspot in Bombay Bazaar, built around serpentine alleys and overcrowded slums. They were counselling a patient with diabetes – and therefore likely to have serious complications due to COVID – when a group of men charged towards them, taking aim with stones and rocks. The women, both in their late twenties, had to make a run for it as the mob hunted them down and chased them out of the neighbourhood. The doctors were puzzled. They had been running field testing camps for several days and nothing like this had ever happened. Later, Trupti thought, maybe it was a result of all the fake news circulating on WhatsApp forwards. 'I'd only seen scenes like this in the movies,' Zakia told me.

COVID was a seismic jolt that cracked open our illusions of civility and social unity and left our fissures exposed. The aftershocks were felt till long after. Hate-mongering prime-time shows pounced on the horrific assault on the female doctors and twisted its narrative into its being about Hindu doctors coming under assault in a Muslim neighbourhood. The friends, who said they are so close that they always ask for the same shifts and the same assignments, dismissed the attempt to use religion to divide them. 'They can give whatever colour they want to; we don't care, we have been the closest of friends for years and none of this will make any difference to our relationship,' Trupti declared, pointing to photographs of them at shared picnics in the sun, afternoons of shopping, cramming for tough exams together and doing all the things that friends who are shaped and formed by shared experiences do. They were not overly concerned by the attempts to drive a wedge between them; they knew that would not happen. But they were unnerved by the ferocity of the mob hatred they had faced for no reason but that they were doctors. They returned to the same neighbourhood the next morning with a police squad. The local qazi apologized too, on behalf of the men who had behaved so egregiously with them. But the scars would take a long time to fade away. 'Perhaps, for the first time in my life, I realized what it means to be scared for my life,' Trupti said.

Over two waves and two cruel summers, India's healthcare workers did not just fight the virus; they waged multiple wars. If prejudice was the enemy in 2020, being unarmed in the battlefield and then being expected to deliver victory was the crisis of 2021.

If beds ran short in the first year, oxygen and drugs were in drastic short supply in the next eruption of the pandemic. Bound by the ethics and standards of the Hippocratic oath, so named after the ancient Greek physician, healthcare workers found their hands tied and their hearts heavy with helplessness. As the health system collapsed, the queues were infinite and the images from inside hospitals horrific. 'It's like being sent to defend yourself in a nuclear war with a lathi,' Mufazzal Lakdawala, a bariatric surgeon by training, who volunteered to be a first responder, told me sardonically. He helmed the COVID field hospital at Mumbai's NSCI Dome, a massive sports facility that usually played host to professional kabaddi tournaments, MTV reality shows and dandiya nights.

Jumbo facilities became an imperative because hospitals across India began to heave and wobble under the force of the first wave.

At Mumbai's KEM Hospital, we met patients who would spend nights on cardboard strips made from empty boxes they carried to the hospital as they awaited their turn to be treated. At Lilavati Hospital, patients spread their sheets and lay down on the lobby floor, right at the entrance. At Sion Hospital, corpses, wrapped in black plastic sheets, were kept side by side on a single stretcher as doctors frantically attended to patients in the same ward. In the emergency section, two patients, both women, were strapped on a bed meant for one. They lay still, seemingly unconscious, their arms by their sides, one in a yellow floral nightie, the other in a pink sari. Instead of a sanitized, pristine and controlled environment, a video of the hospital showed a facility that looked like a crowded railway platform. There were people huddled on the floor, right next to the walls of the premises itself. Makeshift partitions had been created around beds by stringing a plain-coloured sheet to a wheelable stand. On one bed, a relative was helping a patient wear a mask. Even this 1,400-bed hospital – larger than most – was hardly sufficient at the peak of the crisis. Television networks presented these leaked videos as evidence of scandal and callousness.

The dean of Sion Hospital was edged out.

At the front line of battle, this narrative only added insult to injury.

In the war against COVID, it was government hospitals that consistently held the fort and young resident doctors who were the foot soldiers. Decades of neglect and underspending on public health made it impossible for the system to suddenly be battle ready.

Across the street from Sion Hospital's rudimentary and unremarkable yellow-and-grey building, four doctors, all in their early twenties, met me to talk about how demoralized the media reportage had made them.

'This will create an identity crisis for us and the hospitals we work for,' said Dr Rishab, a confident but angry young man. 'If you judge us this harshly, this unfairly for things we cannot control, how will we keep going ahead? The health system in big countries, richer countries like the USA, Italy, has broken down. Why are we pretending it should be any different for us? We are overwhelmed. With these videos, are we trying to create mistrust between the general population and doctors? Do we want them to be scared of coming to the hospital?'

At 0.55 beds for every 1,000 Indians and just 0.66 doctors for every 1,000 people, India should hardly have been surprised at what followed.[14] Essentially, one in every three Indians does not get proper access to a doctor. And this was before COVID. 'Imagine, it has taken a pandemic for us to talk about our health system,' said Akshay, another doctor at Sion. 'Doctors are facing violence from relatives when we can't admit patients. You call us corona warriors, so do you backstab your warriors in the middle of battle?'

Lakdawala walked me through the 'Dome', past high-tech portable ICUs and giant overhead TV screens streaming afternoon melodramas 'as a happy distraction'. We made our way through a maze of giant oxygen cylinders, one for every patient showing serious symptoms. This was year one and oxygen supply had not proven to be a major crisis. Dozens of patients from the Tata Memorial Cancer Hospital had been shifted here too; their autoimmune disorder by definition made them most vulnerable to COVID. It was a sophisticated, contemporary COVID response. But the doctor's optimistic and excited tone at what could be achieved changed when he stopped to consider the most basic of facts. He could procure expensive machines, he could use CCTV cameras to monitor patients, he could build a giant oxygen-generating machine, but he was still short of the most precious commodity of all – medical personnel. For the first time in their history, local train services in Mumbai were suspended, making it impossible for much of the support staff to reach their places of work. But even otherwise, there was a dire shortage of personnel. Lakdawala was now accepting non-medical volunteers to staff in more general roles; he was making video appeals on Instagram for city residents to sign up.

Older doctors, with years of experience, were almost apoplectic with rage at the public attitude towards them, especially at the easy, armchair judgements about how the crisis should be managed.

'People keep asking why we are admitting patients to the lobby of our hospital; where do you want them to go?' asked Jalil

Parkar, a pulmonary specialist at Lilavati Hospital, who is the go-to doctor for the film industry's biggest stars. Dilip Kumar relied on his care till he breathed his last. Unlike many other celebrity doctors, Parkar did not care much about cultivating an image or wearing a veneer. He would often erupt in anger or cry softly. But he always spoke his mind. 'People are coming to us from everywhere, not just the city, but from villages and towns and beyond. They are so scared of collapsing on the way. When they come to the hospital we cannot just push them out. So we treat them where we can, however we can. Temporarily, we are treating them on chairs, even by giving them wheelchairs to sit in – we have created a triage in the lobby – we are also treating those who are forced to lie on the floor because there are no beds. We are doing what we can. But it is an inhuman, desperate situation. Please do not tell me this will get over in a month or even a year. It is such a sorry state of affairs that I barely have words to articulate it. The system is combusting. This is worse than the Second World War.'

Parkar, who is in his early sixties, contracted the infection in early 2020, and though he could have sequestered himself at home citing his age, he was back to ICU duty the moment he was better. 'I felt deeply hurt; even I had a problem getting a bed at first in my own hospital,' he said, recalling the days he spent with his wife, who also tested COVID positive, in the same ward, the couple separated by a sheet. 'I saw death and returned. Till the vaccines came, the truth is even doctors did not know what worked. We started with azithromycin, plasma therapy, moved to tocilizumab, steroids and blood thinners. But we do not know, really did not know.'

Grappling with different shortages from year one to the next, health workers were reaching a point of acute PTSD. 'We are all tired,' said Parkar. 'Our nurses, security staff, technicians – our postgraduate students who are giving their lives because of the shortage of doctors – they are especially tired. This is a wake-up call for all of us. It is very insulting, very humiliating. We are not animals, we are human beings. Please, for God's sake, I am begging you with folded hands, stop this nonsense. What wrong have we done? By admitting patients in our hospital lobby, have we admitted them in a bloody toilet or something? If my hospital has ten storeys, where do you want me to get five more floors from in the middle of a pandemic? Stop sitting behind your laptops and pointing fingers at us. Come to the ground.'

As the first phase of the pandemic appeared to settle down, a new conflict erupted between the government and the Indian Medical Association. Just how many lives of doctors, nurses, ward boys and nurse orderlies had been swept up in the first wave?

There was simply no agreement.

In February 2021, the government informed Parliament that 174 doctors, 116 nurses and 119 other health workers had died from COVID. In the same week, the Indian Medical Association's report placed the number of doctors who had died at 734, including 431 who were general practitioners and the first point of contact for most patients. The association believed the government had shown 'shocking apathy' in refusing to cross-verify data provided to it by the umbrella body of doctors. 'Mortality and morbidity are both being hidden,' alleged Dr R.V. Ashokan, an office bearer with the association. 'Those who have died should be treated as martyrs.' This dispute over just how many health workers were lost to COVID remained unresolved.

Lost in the contestation of claims were the individual

tragedies of health workers claimed by COVID. Not just had we reduced front-line workers to mere statistics; we had failed to even do the maths.

From cemeteries in Chennai to cremation grounds in Delhi, this was the colossal tragedy of India's health workers. Over the next few months, people slowly grew more aware of funeral protocols and thus less scared. But many medical professionals, in particular those down the ranks, suffered silently.

There could be no irony crueller than a health worker who had risked her life for the well-being of COVID patients being unable to find a bed or a hospital willing to treat her when the virus struck her. At Delhi's Nigambodh Ghat, where in the pre-pandemic years VIP politicians were brought for their last rites, two young men stood under the watchful and benevolent eye of a Lord Krishna statue. They were distraught – their mother Seema, the matriarch of their family and a health worker at Lok Nayak Jai Prakash Nayak (LNJP) Hospital, had just died from COVID. They were there to see if they could find a corner to cremate her. But the grounds were overrun with bodies. They had already spent an entire day on their motorcycle, going from funeral home to funeral home in search of a spot where they could say a final farewell to Seema. They had no idea where to look next. Seema, a nurse orderly – support staff to nurses and doctors – had come home from hospital with a stomach ache and a fever one day. Testing for COVID, the RT-PCR swabs that we take for granted today, had not been streamlined yet. At this time, fewer than 500 government laboratories along with 204 private centres were authorised nationwide for lab testing. Which means, in the summer of 2020, India was sorely under-testing. Daily COVID tests for every 1,000 people were 0.08 in India, compared with 1.16 in the US and 1.02 in Italy.[15] During this stage in the pandemic, experts were calling for a tenfold increase in testing. For people like Seema, despite working in a hospital, albeit at the lower end of the hierarchy, access to testing and medical treatment was not a guarantee. At least not at a time when hospitals were running out of oxygenated beds. LNJP was now converted fully into a COVID facility and was not willing to give Seema a bed based on her other symptoms. Her children took her in an autorickshaw from hospital to hospital. They visited eight different centres, including Ambedkar Hospital, B.L. Kapoor Hospital, Dr. Ram Manohar Lohia Hospital (RML), St Stephen's Hospital and, of course LNJP, where she worked at the front line. When one of the hospitals finally agreed to test her, the result was negative. Because of this she was not able to get admission anywhere. But Seema had died from COVID. That fact, however, could only be ascertained after it was too late. It was found in her post-mortem. By then Seema had died on the road, in the arms of her sons and nephew, at just fifty. Her son, standing in front of a faded yellow wall on which a graffiti scrawl asked people to be careful and stand two metres apart, proudly pulled out his mother's identity card for me to see. He had shown the same card at the gates of more than half a dozen hospitals and clinics, in the hope that it would move them into responding. That did not happen. Now they were being shunted around between multiple cremation grounds? 'Are we animals?' he asked me.

Over the course of the two waves of the pandemic, the stigma against health workers receded, but a tornado of shortages hit hospitals and torpedoed them yet again. Doctors and nurses were now vulnerable like never before.

In the months of April and May 2021, ICUs became war zones.

In Mumbai, inside the ICU of the privately run SRV Hospital, Dr Rupkatha, the intensivist on duty, said she was short of everything – drugs, beds, oxygen, tocilizumab and, yes, even doctors. In the same ward, her colleague Dr Nida's mother was a patient, but she had to emotionally dissociate from her and attend to other patients. In Bengaluru, inside the ICU of HBS Hospital, Dr Taha Mateen said he could hardly bear to see how young some of the patients were. 'It's death upon death; pain upon pain.' In Surat's Civil Hospital there was a line at the pharmacy that ran at least a mile long. At first, I thought it consisted of the relatives of patients admitted in the wards. But I was shocked to find that the line was made up almost entirely of healthcare workers, including many young doctors from smaller nursing homes and hospitals, who had come to the government-run facility in search of remdesivir. They would queue up at the crack of dawn to get a spot in the line and a chance at getting the controversial broad-spectrum antiviral medication before it ran out for that day. From finding oxygen vendors to drugs that were either in short supply or had been swallowed up by a black market now became the job of either health workers or patients.

This was the other crisis for India's doctors in the second wave. There was no evidence-based medical regimen that they could deploy. Though the vaccines were now available as a preventive, their slow roll-out meant it was too late to vaccinate the country out of the surge. Therapeutic interventions, save some nascent use of monoclonal antibodies, had not yet been approved. A word-of-mouth medical 'package' had emerged, which included ivermectin, the anti-parasite drug mostly used as a deworming pill for horses and livestock, the steroid dexamethasone, a course of standard antibiotics, the antiviral drug fabiflu and expensive injections such as remdesivir and tocilizumab. Remdesivir acquired an urban legend status right through the second wave, though in November 2020, WHO clearly advised against its use for COVID treatment. The use of ivermectin was so widespread in India that even when its own parent pharmaceutical company urged for it not to be used it continued to be used for months on end till the government dropped it from the protocol in June 2021. By this time the second wave had begun to recede. Because doctors were still grappling with the great unknown, the lack of clarity in medical treatment only added to the fraught environment at hospitals and the breakdown of trust between doctors and patients.

Viral videos from hospitals across the country showed families of patients coming to blows with staff on being denied a bed or in the aftermath of a death. 'In this war, I am ready to lose my life to COVID in trying to save a patient,' said Mufazzal Lakdawala to me. 'But I am not ready to die at the hands of an irate relative because the government's infrastructure failed. That is the story of every doctor today.'

The mental health of young doctors who spent long hours in the ICU started showing signs of fraying.

One day, on her way back home from hospital at the peak of the surge in May 2021, Dr Trupti Gilada, whose baby girl Muskan was born during the first wave, felt she just couldn't breathe any more. She felt the panic well up in waves. She parked her car to one side, leaned back in the seat, took a deep breath and took out her phone. She wanted to film something that she could share in her family WhatsApp group. She still had her hospital scrubs on, including a thin blue shower-cap-like elastic cap covering her head. As she began to give an account of what was happening in Mumbai, the tears ran down her chin from beneath her spectacles. 'I have never felt this helpless, this *lachar*,' she wept, using the Hindi word for powerlessness. 'If any of you think you have not got COVID for a year and so you are safe you are wrong. We have a thirty-five-year-old on a ventilator and we can't help him. We are having to manage patients at home because we have no room in the hospitals.' The video spread on the internet like a forest fire, leaving no one untouched because of the searing authenticity of this front line doctor who was also a new mother. Later, reflecting on the meltdown she experienced, she said, 'There isn't any caregiver at the front line who hasn't had some emotional breakdown. It's a mix of frustration at what could have been prevented, helplessness with patients and fear of what may happen next. One of the primary emotions is anger. We had a year to prepare for this moment, to roll out vaccines, to make sure we weren't short of ICU beds again. Yes, this [the Delta variant] is a more lethal strain but there was a lull of four months. We could have been ready. But we thought the war had already been won. We are to blame, both the government and we, the people.'

But in the end, for soldiers who had signed up for the battle, it was really the details that no one had bothered asking about that were momentous.

Like the nurse in Pune who told me that she felt shattered because when she went home after duty her children would no longer let her feed them. Because she spent long hours in a sweaty PPE, the kids said she smelt of burnt plastic.

Or the doctor at Safdarjung Hospital who was pregnant and whispered to me that she was terrified that she would miscarry the child from the sheer anxiety of her job.

For women, in particular, the costs were distinct.

No one had sought to think, for instance, what might happen

to nurses or doctors menstruating in a PPE kit, which was made in such a way that it was a single, airless sheath of plastic draping the body from head to toe. You could not use the bathroom while wearing it, leave alone change a sanitary pad or tampon. I may never have paid attention to this detail were it not for the fact that every time I had to wear a PPE to report from inside a COVID ward or hospital, I would find that I was sick for hours afterwards. Not just would I go racing outside into the open air as soon as the assignment was complete, stripping off the smelly blue plastic, I would also feel weak for hours afterwards, often emotionally brittle and quick to tears too. For someone who has long been exposed to hazardous situations in the line of work, this was a highly unusual experience for me and I did not want to give it too much importance. I met Yogita Bagad in Mumbai. No one could accuse a nurse who had battled Ajmal Kasab and rescued new mothers from COVID of being less than tough. So when Yogita told me how the PPE kit seemed to cut off the oxygen supply to her brain, leaving her nearly asphyxiated, prone to panic and especially weak during her period, my own reactions suddenly made much more sense to me.

Yogita, draped in a white PPE, looking like an astronaut about to set foot on the moon, held her arm forward for me to see. 'Look at how the sweat gathers and piles up in one place under the plastic,' she said, opening up about the palpitations that left her feeling mentally disoriented and confused. Her face was hidden behind layers of protective gear – face shields, special glasses – but the consequence was that she was gasping for breath and found it difficult to speak for long stretches. The suffocating suit left her entire body drenched in sweat. And while on her period this meant that '. . . my private parts have a fungal infection, my body and head hurt and I feel like I am going to faint. But I tell myself, I am here for my patients. This is my duty. I have to manage somehow.'

The nurse who dealt with an Ajmal Kasab attack – and then with COVID for two years in a row – was now preparing for a third wave and a new variant.

In Chennai, at the end of the second wave, Dr Simon Hercules's family finally got some overdue emotional closure. His body was exhumed and reburied at the Kilpauk cemetery, as per his dying wish. But not before his wife Anandi had to fight a year-long battle in the Madras High Court.

In December 2021, the Indian Medical Association (IMA) provided a list of 1,700 doctors to the government who it said had died as a result of the pandemic.

Tragically, stepping into 2022, no doctor believed that the roster of death would end with the year gone by.

During the two years of the pandemic, what happened to those who suffered from tuberculosis (TB), cancer, kidney disease and other pulmonary disorders? As hospital systems got overtaken by the pandemic in both 2020 and 2021, the fatalities from other infectious diseases have mounted. India will not be able to meet its stated goal of ending TB in 2025. In April 2020, as the first wave surged, one million fewer children got the BCG vaccine (which prevents severe TB) than just three months earlier, in January 2020. And half of all new cancer cases likely went untreated. None of the fatalities that may have been accelerated as a result of no medical intervention have been formally documented or added to the pandemic's official toll.

4

Five Girls and a Funeral

They carried their father on their slender shoulders, distributing the weight of the body on the stretcher made from bamboo and leaves between the five of them. At five years old, Jyoti, the littlest among them, really just ran alongside the four older girls.

It was left to Kajal, the eldest, who was nineteen, to lead the way and hold her grieving family together. Wearing a printed red-and-black salwar kurta, her hand wrapped tightly around the bamboo pole, she wept as she walked towards the funeral pyre. Her sisters, in T-shirts and loosely fitted cotton pyjamas with elastic waistbands, took their cue from her, but were probably too young to process the enormity of what they were witnessing.

In Aligarh, in western Uttar Pradesh, this made for a radical image. It was still not common for women to attend burials and cremations, leave alone perform the last rites.

But Sanjay Gupta – a teaseller who sold over-sweet milky chai in chipped glasses from a hole-in-the-wall shack propped up by rickety wooden planks – had no sons. His death from TB may not have been noticed were it not for his daughters. Two of them had shaved off their hair in keeping with the Hindu ritual of mundan, a mourning custom typically followed by boys on the death of a close relative. A third had a huge turban tied around her small head. Their quiet rebellion drew attention to what would otherwise have been one more invisible death slipping anonymously through the COVID cracks.

It was 5 April 2020. The cumulative count of those infected with COVID was 3,588. And that day itself at least 1,400 Indians, Sanjay Gupta among them, died from TB.

But no one was paying any attention. The Indian mind space was so consumed by COVID and its health system so preoccupied with it that other infectious diseases, many of them fatal, barely caused a blip.

Blue-and-orange tarpaulin sheets were now thrown like a shroud over the small store where Sanjay once sold tea. Across the road from it the family gathered in a barely furnished room in which a couple of brown plastic chairs were placed against a faded wall, now more grey than white. Two steel vessels and a single gas cylinder for meals sat across from the bed, which was the only other piece of furniture in the room. On a small ledge, a single earthen diya sat alongside a bottle of liver tonic, prescribed to their father for strength. The diya, with its burnt-out wick, had been lit by the girls a day after their father's death. The prime minister had asked the country for '9 minutes at 9', a rallying cry of national unity at a time of crisis. The Gupta family had also purchased a handful of clay diyas and kerosene to join millions of their fellow citizens in a symbolic show of support for health workers at the COVID front line. Instead, they found themselves organizing a funeral.

But the girls lit the diyas nevertheless.

When Sanjay's condition deteriorated, the family took him

to the government district hospital, but there were no doctors available to see him. After a couple of wasted trips, his brother Narendra appealed to doctors at a small private hospital to examine him. But such was the paranoia about attending to patients without their first being tested for COVID that he was turned away. The family knew they were losing time. As his condition worsened, the daughters tried to get an ambulance to rush their father to hospital. But calls to two different helplines drew a blank. They lost two critical hours. By the time they managed to get him to the government hospital they discovered most of the wards had been blocked for COVID patients. The TB specialists were not on duty either. The compounder prescribed some basic medicine for Sanjay's fever and sent him home. That same day, he died.

Even before the pandemic, only 26 per cent of district government hospitals met the government-mandated norms on the positioning of doctors.[16] In a post-COVID ecosystem, even those standards collapsed.

Because it was the beginning of the pandemic, panic was pushing everyone who tested positive into hospital. At this stage, even doctors were urging those with symptoms to not delay hospital intervention. Entire super-speciality medical centres were being turned into COVID-only facilities, rendering them redundant and off limits for other patients. Some of this was inevitable for that stage of the pandemic.

But it was clearly a mistake.

Those with mild to moderate symptoms should have been encouraged to isolate at home, leaving hospitals and doctors free for other patients. Like in actual battle, field hospitals, possibly built by the military, could have been one way forward. But even when giant sporting stadiums and venues for music concerts were repurposed as temporary hospitals, for many months at a stretch the medical system remained inaccessible to those grappling with other forms of illness.

This was despite the fact that TB alone had claimed 0.45 million lives in 2018 in India, which accounted for 30 per cent of all TB deaths globally.[17] These did not include the deaths of patients that remained undetected, mortalities that were never notified or people who may have died as a result of misdiagnosis. It is these 'missing' cases that have got doctors extremely worried about the grave setback to India's aspiration to be tuberculosis-free by 2025.

Between March and June 2019, 860,787 TB cases were notified in India by both the public and private sector. Those numbers dropped to 465,051 for the same period in 2020, three months that overlapped with the national lockdown.[18] That's a drop of 46 per cent. India wasn't the only country, of course, to grapple with this phenomenon. Worldwide, there was a dip of 1.3 million reported TB cases. India accounted for 41 per cent of these.[19]

Madhu Pai, a passionate global advocate for public health equity, trained at Vellore in India before he became a professor at McGill University in Canada, was categorical about the devastating consequences of overlooking other diseases during the pandemic. 'Due to the COVID-19 pandemic, lockdowns and disruptions of health services, TB care in India has been seriously compromised, with more than a 20 per cent drop in the number of TB patients notified during 2020 (compared to previous years). The drop is much higher during 2021, since India had a devastating Delta wave crisis. India will not be able to end TB by 2025. In fact, it will take years to recover from this damage and will require massive investments in the TB programme by the government, and greater investment in health itself. India continues to underinvest in health and the consequences were visible during this pandemic,' he told me.

It was almost as if the virus was imposing hierarchical privilege over the sickness pecking order.

The pandemic pushed everyone else out of the health system.

And, as always, it was the poor who suffered the most.

'*Allah tala inko bacha la, kisi bhi tarah bacha lo,*' (Allah, please save him somehow, anyhow.) implored Nayema, the tears running down her face, her hands folded in submission to a higher power that she believed had decided to punish her. Her husband, Mohammad Ishtiaq, sat by her side, wearing just a vest. They leaned against a sordid pink wall pockmarked by grey soot, huddling together on a thin mattress placed on the floor of the single room that was their home.

They were surrounded by papers – prescriptions, hospital discharge slips, bills and an oncologist's reference for chemotherapy.

Ishtiaq's face was entirely disfigured. Oral cancer had swollen his right cheek into a giant, infected balloon that appeared to float over the horizon of his shoulder. When we met him he was in excruciating pain, a physical trauma so visceral that it made him writhe and weep. Like his wife, he too folded his hands and pleaded: 'Help me.'

Through tears, his wife Nayema told us how Ishtiaq had been unable to sleep for days altogether. At night he would flail his arms about, kick his legs, turn from side to side and scream in pain.

A labourer who lived off project-driven daily earnings, Ishtiaq had been operated on at the capital's Guru Tegh Bahadur Hospital in January 2020. His cancer had metastasized and a growth had been removed from part of his shoulder too. He had been referred to a cancer speciality hospital for chemotherapy, but since the lockdown had been imposed he had not managed to get even one session to zap his galloping, cannibalizing cells.

Nayema and Ishtiaq spread out their documents like forensic detectives on a case. There were X-rays and endless lists of drugs and a count of the number of hospitals and doctors they had tried to visit or meet. 'Sometimes they say there is no doctor available. Sometimes they say, go get a COVID test first and sometimes they make some other excuse. They are lying, they are lying,' said Ishtiaq, his helplessness manifesting as rage.

Every night his wife and two children would sit around Ishtiaq, hold his hand, put cold towels on his head, massage his head and do anything to distract him from the acute and violent discomfort he was experiencing. Because one side of his face had grown so large, it caused him pain to lie down. He would spend the nights sitting up, clasping his wife's hand for strength.

'If we had money, we would go to a private hospital,' Ishtiaq said, crestfallen. 'But things are so bad, we barely have food to eat.'

Their daughter, the eldest of three, had completed her schooling and aspired to get a college degree. But she had to surrender her plans for further education because of the situation at home. She now stitched clothes to add a few rupees to the house kitty.

If 1,400 Indians die from TB every day, just as many lives are claimed by cancer daily.

But the pandemic had stripped away the pretence of equality among citizens when it came to the Right to Life. If you thought of the virus as an MRI machine, it had scanned the insides of the

Indian health system to reveal the uncomfortable, inconvenient, bare-boned truth: Indian lower-income groups, dependent on publicly funded medical facilities, had nowhere to go and no one to turn to.

The first wave was especially damaging because doctors, nurses and the government were still feeling their way through the maze of the crisis, their vision blurry and senses inflamed. When hospitals were not taken over entirely by COVID patients, they would be sealed and shut down the moment there was a positive case. The 180-bed Delhi Cancer Hospital closed its gates after eighteen staffers tested positive; Mumbai's Wockhardt facility was shuttered after more than three dozen staff members got COVID. These were still early days and isolation protocols were not fully understood. There was still the mistaken belief that the virus leapfrogged from surface to surface and room to room. The utopian idea of 'zero COVID' was still being pursued. Just like housing societies and factories that would immediately and unscientifically be cordoned off and barricaded even if there was a single positive case in an otherwise giant complex, hospitals too were treated in the same way.

The result: COVID patients often did not find a hospital bed and those with other grave illnesses almost never did; too often they were not even able to get basic medical intervention. Often, this would have fatal consequences. The pandemic death toll does not even begin to count the thousands, likely hundreds of thousands, of lives that were lost across two years from illnesses other than COVID, but as a direct consequence of decisions taken during the pandemic. If an Indian citizen died from kidney disease or cancer or TB because he or she could not get a doctor, medicine or an ambulance, should they not be considered a casualty of the COVID years? Tragically, leave alone counting them in the pandemic death toll, even their stories were barely told.

R.V. Pundhir's children have a recording of probably the last time he ever spoke to anyone on the telephone. It might even be the last time he spoke at all, they say. It is a clip of a phone call he made to the hospital to try and convince them that he was in desperate need of his scheduled dialysis session. '*Bahut pareshan hoon, bahut bechaini hai,*' he says in the recording, talking about his pain and restlessness, his voice halting between syllables, the verbal equivalent of a physical limp. '*Kisi tarah meri dialysis karva dijiye,*' (Please help me get my dialysis done) he says, nearly crying, pleading for the intervention that would have flushed out toxins from his body, a job that his disease-ridden kidneys could no longer perform on their own.

This was in Agra, the world capital of romance, where the streets had been scrubbed and the lamp posts painted and polished for the visit of Donald Trump just a couple of months ago. Posters for English tutorials, the best butter chicken and engineering entrance exams – the staple hand-printed flyers in pink and white normally pasted randomly across public walls in the smaller towns of India – had all been taken down. On the day I met the family of R.V. Pundhir, multicoloured murals of Hanuman and Ganesha and slogans of India Rising dotted the landscape. The city looked dressed up and joyous even in lockdown.

The grief of broken families was obscured and needed to be excavated.

In the Neerav Nikunj neighbourhood, in a dreary lane where single-storeyed houses with common walls stood in a row, there was one home where a white bed sheet was spread out on the floor of the driveway, generally used to park the car. On the floor, women sat huddled together, consoling each other as they wept. Their cries of pain came from the gut, tearing through the eerie silence of the curfewed evening. They were sitting around a small wooden table dressed with a white lace tablecloth bearing a framed photograph of R.V. Pundhir. 'I am left without any support, *main besahara ho gayee,*' his wife Radha kept repeating, in a daze.

On Friday, 17 April 2020, R.V. Pundhir was slated to get one of his two weekly sessions of dialysis at the private Patni Medical Centre. He had been treated there for chronic kidney disease for six years. But there was a new prerequisite: a COVID negative test. Remember, this was still the first couple of months of the crisis and testing was not yet ubiquitous or even allowed across private laboratories and hospitals. The waiting line to be swabbed was long, and to get the results took even longer. The next morning, Pundhir's son, Akshay, took his father to the district hospital, where the queue ran a mile long and suspected COVID patients stood shoulder to shoulder with others who were mandated to get a test. His father's blood pressure was falling and Askhay had to cradle him in his arms to provide him support. His father sat in a plastic chair while Akshay stood in line instead. The test done, they returned home hoping for the best. On Sunday, Pundhir's BP had fallen and he felt he was sinking. The children dialled the 108 helpline for an ambulance. A couple of hours passed and there was still no vehicle available. So, taking the help of their neighbour, they bundled him into the back of their car and drove to three different hospitals, the government-run S.N. Medical College and two private facilities. All three declined admission without evidence of the patient being COVID negative. The family pleaded for basic emergency intervention, a blood pressure machine and oxygen support. They filmed shaky phone videos everywhere they went of resigned, laconic medical workers and security guards asking them to leave, in the hope that the fear of being recorded for posterity would evoke a different response. It had no impact; Pundhir died a few hours later. The COVID tests finally came, the next morning, on Monday. He had tested negative.

The singular fixation on COVID by the health system, the lockdown restrictions, the shortage of doctors and medical staff and the mismanagement of available health infrastructure have created massive gaps both in the response to other diseases and in the documentation of data.

India, which accounts for one in every four cases of TB globally, for instance, saw a 60 per cent decline in the number of cases registered in the month of April 2020 from the corresponding numbers in 2019. Otherwise, the country reports 2.64 million new cases every year. The target for India was to eliminate TB by 2025, five years ahead of the United Nations-set Sustainable Development Goals. Some epidemiologists are worried that the steep stumble in recording cases – which effectively means hundreds of thousands of Indians did not get treatment in time – could set back the country's TB programme by a decade or more. Nor do we have any precise empirical measure of how many more deaths this means.

For already immunocompromised cancer patients the pandemic has been especially traumatic and dangerous. A study across forty-one cancer centres reveals an untold humanitarian crisis. Between March and May 2020, there was a 54 per cent reduction in the number of cancer cases registered – which means half of all new cancer cases in India were possibly untreated. Hospital admissions took a severe hit with a 36 per cent drop. Outpatient chemotherapy was impacted as well, with a 37 per cent reduction. Life-saving surgeries fell by 49 per cent. And, most worrying of all, even routine screenings either stopped entirely or were at 25 per cent of their usual number at the majority of the centres.[20] The effectiveness of cancer treatment almost always depends on how early you catch it. We simply have no precise count of how many cancer complications and deaths were hastened because of the absence of timely intervention.

Over open sewage drains and past rickety street carts that have neither vendors nor wares is the neighbourhood of Bhalswa Dairy, a slum colony in north-east Delhi, where exposed electricity wires are bunched and tied together across slender lanes. On a hot June afternoon, the local banana seller was asleep as flies hovered over fruit no one had any money to buy. Some men sat around under the shade of an awning, while all around them mounds of cement and rubble piled up at abandoned construction sites. In this slum colony, where most residents are factory workers or daily-wage labour, up the steep staircase of one of the pocket-sized plots, a tiny kitchen opened up into a single room. Beads framed the entry to the room instead of a door, and behind them was the blur of a woman resting on her side.

Another woman with short cropped hair met us with folded hands and bowed head. Help us, she said quietly.

Mamata, twenty-six, has stage-three breast cancer. Dressed in a printed floral nightie, she lay writhing in pain, just below a calendar cut-out print of two tigers painted in vivid orange and blue. On a ledge nailed to the wall a few metres above were a couple of mugs for tea, steel vessels and tumblers, and plastic boxes to store odds and ends. Nailed to the side of her bed were mounted clasps in which a bunch of spoons were displayed. Her friend Suchitra, the woman who greeted us at the door, and whom Mamata calls her sister, was wearing pyjamas and a T-shirt printed with the insignia of warrior games. She was fussing over the woman, whose survival had come to be the mission of her life.

As Suchitra stroked Mamata's hair, gently pulling back the strands of black falling on her blue surgical mask, Mamata told us that she was asked to leave Delhi's LNJP Hospital a week after being admitted for treatment. The public hospital was mandated to convert into a COVID-only facility and Mamata was asked to find an alternative arrangement. A kind doctor told Mamata she was so weak that a gust of wind would knock her down. He advised that she may have no option but to isolate herself at home. But it hasn't been easy. As the cancer metastasizes Mamata had been grappling with a shooting pain, one that rushed through her bloodstream in sharp, sudden bursts. 'Please, dear God,' she broke down, 'either allow me to live well or let me die.'

Watching her collapse, Suchitra was unable to remain stoic. She folded her hands again. 'Can you help us get to the hospital, any hospital? Do something, but get us admitted to hospital.'

Suchitra earned ₹5,000 working as contract labour in a small factory that made coloured threads. But she lost her job after she was compelled to take long absences from work to look after Mamata, who hadn't been able to go out and earn a living for the past year. Another neighbour left cooked meals of lentils and rice a few times a week and helped them just about get by. The day she didn't send food, Suchitra went to the neighbourhood school and came back with leftover food from the midday meal served for students from the economically weaker sections. Since the imposition of the lockdown, the school had gone online, closing one more avenue of sustenance for them. 'I have heard AIIMS [All India Institutes of Medical Sciences] is very good . . .'

Mamata's voice trailed off softly, as her thoughts appeared to wander away from her body. The painkillers helped for a couple of hours, but then, she said, she started flipping like a fish with pain. Before falling asleep, she had a final question to ask of us.

'Will I live?'

The sentence repeated most often in media commentary through the pandemic – that the virus is an equalizing force leaping across the divides of class, caste and gender – is also the biggest lie of our times. As a domestic worker who earned a living washing vessels and rolling rotis in the swanky apartment buildings of Mumbai told me, the rich brought the virus to India on a plane and it is the poor who are suffering on the streets. Every subterranean inequality that was otherwise too inconvenient to dig up from the quarries of extreme privilege was exposed by the landslide impact of the crisis. Across the trench lines of gender, men fared better than women. At the bottom of the social hierarchy, Dalits did worse than so-called upper castes. The cities were islands of privilege in contrast to the villages that were nudged out of public recall. And in a country where the rich already outlive the poor by an average of seven and a half years, these two years reinforced every single inequity in the healthcare system. Even before the pandemic, poor households spent nearly 15 per cent of their monthly income on healthcare compared to the richest households who spent less than 1 per cent of their wealth on the same.[21] Now there was just bewilderment, hopelessness and resignation as the poor got pushed around from hospital to hospital, carrying little scraps of paper in faded folders, thrust in their hands by doctors too overworked to have the time to explain anything to them.

These were men and women who waited long hours to get a rushed appointment with a harassed, overworked, health worker who would scribble out an advised line of treatment and rush them along to attend to the next patient. Often their prescription slips felt like communiques in an alien language, so much so that they were not even fully cognizant of how bleak the prognosis was. COVID multiplied these inequities. Even a few hours outside any state-run hospital in India threw up tragedy after tragedy, till there were too many to count.

And so it was that Rajesh, a pavement dweller, found himself outside the gates of LNJP Hospital. Security guards were now like bouncers at a coveted bar, their effectiveness directly proportional to how many people they could turn away from the wrought-iron gates. A black-and-white chequered scarf was wrapped around Rajesh's face though this was the middle of summer. He was a thin, almost undernourished man who carried a giant cloth bag filled with documents and little scraps of paper. When he dropped the makeshift mask around his face, people stared and then quickly recoiled and looked away. His upper lip was swollen to the size of a balloon; his chin had a protrusion as well. There were blobs of pus marks on the inflamed portions. He was standing around somewhat aimlessly, unsure of what he should do next after being told that the hospital, now a fully COVID facility, could not allow him in. He did not even comprehend that he had cancer. When I asked him about his ailment, he thrust a huge file in our direction and asked me to look. A few months ago the doctors at the hospital had diagnosed him with oral cancer. Rajesh had an appointment to collect some subsidized medicines from the hospital. 'I am an illiterate man,' Rajesh said. 'I don't understand any of this. But where do I go now?'

Once again, the absence of clear and effective communication – even old-style messages on radio and the public broadcaster may have worked – around what people should do and where they should turn to if they were ill from reasons other than COVID, led to poor families being shunted around from hospital to hospital. There was Farzana, whose one-year-old boy Saad had an enlarged heart, standing goggle-eyed and helpless outside LNJP hospital. She and her husband, a driver, had been summarily sent away from the Chacha Nehru Children's Hospital, which had no cardiologists or an echocardiogram machine. They asked the doctors if they could get a parcha, a scrap of something, that may open the doors for them at another facility. But they were told they'd just have to try their luck. Saad, in a printed flowery pyjama suit, was finding it tough to breathe. This was the third hospital that had asked them to leave. He had been brought here on the back of a motorcycle, but there was an added problem; they had already used up the money they had to fill the tank of the bike. Farzana's husband had been laid off as businesses shut during the lockdown, so there was no steady source of income.

Then there was seven-year-old Ranadip who was a patient of thalassemia, a blood disorder because of which the body is unable to produce enough haemoglobin. The child needed two blood transfusions a month. His mother Parvati worked as a labourer at construction sites, earning a daily wage of a couple of hundred rupees when she got work. Now the money has dried up. Ranadip has been coming here since he was six months old and first diagnosed; this is the one government hospital his mother knew and was familiar with. The hospital advised them to take a chance at another facility at the other end of the city. But that day, they had no money to spare. They decided to go home and start the battle anew the next morning.

Others waited it out on the pavement, right on the road. Some held their heads in their hands, some collapsed in tears under the weight of anxiety and fear and some just stared vacantly into space, wondering what they may do next. Public transport had been suspended; many had walked here. It would be a long walk back.

The lockdown, the poverty, the absence of anyone to talk to or be guided by outside hospitals, the missing administration and the way entire establishments were taken over for COVID created nothing short of a medical catastrophe.

The outpatient department at AIIMS in the capital has always had more patients than it can handle. An average of 15,000 people come here every day, from far-flung corners of the country, in the hope of subsidized medical treatment. AIIMS, which is by far the hospital of choice, even for powerful politicians, is considered the best medical brain trust in the country. Its director, Randeep Guleria, was chosen by the government to steer the COVID response. But as COVID swept through India, even AIIMS was forced to put up white conical tents on the road outside its gates, with collapsible cots placed in single file, to accommodate as many as possible in one shelter. Men, women and children from some of the most remote parts of India waited here, almost in vain. Some had in fact been asked to leave the hospital and make way for those who had COVID and would need it more. But many had not recovered enough to be able to go back home. Shrikant, a brick worker from Buxar in Bihar, had already dipped into his savings to bring his wife Lalan Devi and their small daughter to Delhi. Lalan Devi had a persistent, unbearable abdominal ache and needed surgery to remove a kidney stone. They had been in Delhi for four months awaiting their turn. She finally got a hospital bed, only to be told that she would have to vacate it. If they went back to Bihar it would be difficult and too expensive to return again. And so they waited, like countless other Indians, for the hospital system to make room for them.

In May 2020, the 'Stop TB' Partnership predicted that a three-month lockdown followed by a ten-month recovery period, in which full medical services were restored, would still mean an additional 500,000 TB-related deaths between 2020 and 2025.

But the recovery never came.

And the dead may never be counted.

Seventy-three per cent of elderly people in India believe their families treated them worsened during the pandemic. Not just were India's elders the most physically vulnerable; the lockdown created severe mental and emotional challenges by pushing them into much lonelier lives. Those who lived alone suffered in particular. And then there were those who were abandoned.

5

Leelawati and the Loneliness of the Elderly

Her slender frame was wrapped in a slippery polyester orange sari offset by a print of muddy brown flowers. Her thinning grey hair was tied neatly into a knot at the nape of her neck. She wore black plastic slippers with a flimsy toe strap, just slightly visible from underneath the pleats of her sari, as she sat hunched over on the pavement steps outside the closed gates of Mumbai's Bandra railway station.

She was crying softly.

Her name was Leelawati. She was seventy years old.

It was the month of May in 2020.

She held on tight to a cloth bag and a packet of Parle glucose biscuits.

I was at the station chronicling the flight of migrant workers from the cities of India. After more than two months of a national lockdown that included the shutdown of public transport, special trains — for labourers who had otherwise been walking hundreds of kilometres to their villages — were finally operational. But there was always a frantic scrum of people at stations across India, looking to escape to what they imagined would be the safety of home. A rumour had spread that today was the last scheduled train out of Mumbai and there was a relentless flood of people who had come to the station in hope.

Out on the road, across from the platform, men, women and children sat huddled together on their haunches, balancing their weight with acrobatic perfection. Others squatted on the low-rise pavement. They were busy talking animatedly among themselves.

No one paid any attention to the old lady or her solitude.

When we made a few inquiries to see if anyone might know her from their neighbourhoods or shanties, people shrugged indifferently. Everyone had too many of their own crises – debt, death, and the desperation to make it out of a city where every source of income had run dry.

I approached Leelawati tentatively, flopping on the floor beside her. Through her inchoate tears she managed to mutter something about hunger and food. A small group of samaritans had distributed cardboard boxes of food to the waiting labourers, stocked with a banana, samosa and a tetrapack of fruit juice.

I urged her to take one.

She pulled down her hospital-green cloth mask and focused intently but quietly on the food. She had not eaten for a full day, sitting by herself at the station. But she thought it was prudent to save half a samosa or at least a piece of fruit for later. She did not have money to buy any food so she was storing it away.

Like everyone else, Leelawati Kedarnath Dube wanted to get on a train. But there was a problem. She wasn't sure of her destination. She had nowhere to go.

She spoke with a soft lisp from having lost all her teeth.

Wrinkles framed her tiny black eyes. A tiny metallic nose pin, rust coloured from decades of living, gleamed in the hot summer sun. Her cheeks were pinched thin, her frame was diminutive and she seemed malnourished and weak. Through intermittent sobs she explained that she had come to Mumbai when her son had suddenly taken ill. Her other son had put her on a train before the pandemic broke and had sent her to nurse him back to health. Now, after the lockdown – she called it 'blackdown' – 'he pushed me and threw me out'.

Her son had a drinking problem, she said. He had turned violent and had asked her to leave. '*Chaar bar maara,*' (He hit me four times) she said, holding up her hand to show me where her son had hit her. For a few seconds we sat uncomfortably in silence.

Then she trembled slightly and carried on speaking. '*Kya karti.* What could I do? *Maar khayee.*'

Her son pushed her out of the house and said, 'Just get out, I don't care, beg if you have to.'

As she wept, I did not know how to console her or how to help her.

I reached out and put one blue-gloved hand to her face, clumsily trying to wipe her tears.

She took my hand and held it.

'*Ek paisa nahin hai.*' (I don't have a single penny.)

She did not have enough money for the train fare. She had walked to the station, stopping every couple of kilometres to ask for directions. 'I thought I would beg my way on to the train, maybe ask people for money at the station. *Bheek mangte hue kahin to pahunch jaoongi.*'

Leelawati was a widow; none of her other children wanted her either. '*Aadmi nahin hai na, isliye . . .*' Her voice trailed off into more sobs as she wondered whether she had been abandoned because she no longer had a man in her life.

Trying to bolster her spirits I muttered something fatuous about how a woman did not have to feel incomplete without a man's support in today's day and age. But what may have otherwise been worthy and true was entirely academic and useless for this moment. She nodded in agreement and then said, '*Main aisi waisi aurat nahin hoon; main bahut seedhi-saadhi hoon.*' She was keen for me to know that she was a simple woman.

She wanted to get to Delhi somehow, the city where she had once lived with her husband. 'I have another son there, but he doesn't want me either. None of my five children want me. No one wants me. They all say I am *paagal*, they call me mad. Do I look mad to you?' she asked me.

Leelawati was crying copiously now.

I leaned forward and hugged her tight. We sat there, at the gates of a railway station, a seventy-year-old and a forty-nine-year-old, strangers locked in an embrace that was counterintuitive to the social distancing norms of the time but a reminder of why the tactile connection between humans mattered so much.

Many institutions failed to work as they should have during this pandemic. And while we spoke a lot about the government, the Opposition, the Election Commission, the police, the courts and the media, there is one that we did not deconstruct – the institution of family.

Leelawati held out a small cardboard box with a silver foil covering to show me how she had been managing for food. It was a half-eaten plate of dry khichdi. '*Nahin roungee*,' (I won't cry) she would tell herself every few minutes and then collapse in a heap of sorrow. 'My husband was a very nice man. Now, just because I am ageing, my children don't want me. So what if I am old?'

Of all the challenges that the pandemic had thrown up, this one was the most overlooked – the loneliness, destitution and abandonment of India's elderly. At 140 million, India has the second largest elderly population in the world. Compared with Western nations, where rambling and giant families have atomized into smaller and smaller units, as Indians we have always prided ourselves on being defined by a sense of community. The idea of pushing our parents into a care home would still be anathema to most. And, though urban living and gated communities have chipped away at the idea of a 'colony, where neighbours are the extended family and the elderly meet over tea and chatter in the common park', we still see ourselves as a fiercely interconnected, interdependent and informal culture. Respect for the elderly is hardwired into us. We fold our hands before them; we instinctively bend down to touch their feet and get their blessings.

Of all the people I met over two years of reporting on COVID, none struck quite as much of a chord as the story of Leelawati did. Once we had placed her plight in the public domain, that single image threw open the floodgates. Perhaps, in Leelawati's plight we saw both our worst fears and our best sides. In her we imagined our own parents, the guilt we felt for falling short, the fears we had about our own age. God forbid this would ever be our mother.

Or worse – us.

All around Leelawati sat workers desperate to get home, somehow, anyhow. And here was an elderly lady, in the twilight of her life, who had no notion of home any longer. Even if we found a way to get her on a train to Delhi, where would she go,

I asked her gently, simultaneously thinking of old-age homes I could get in touch with. '*Koi baat nahin, beta. Dilli mein bheekh mangungi.* (Don't worry, child. I'll survive by begging in Delhi.) Anything, even begging, is better than being here and being thrashed by my own son. I would have preferred to find a way to earn a living. But I am seventy now and I don't have the strength to do too much physical work. *Kya karoon?*'

Ironically, by the end of our conversation it was Leelawati who was consoling me. 'Don't cry because of me, I will feel terrible,' she said, in a tone of grandmother-like admonishing love. 'I am thinking of my husband. I am missing him, [Leelawati was married to an ironworker from Uttar Pradesh] and so I am feeling sad. *Par himmat rakhoongi.*' (But I won't give up.)

In a survey, 73 per cent of the elderly population said they believe attitudes towards them worsened during the lockdown and the second wave. Among these, 61 per cent said deteriorating interpersonal relationships were responsible for incidences of abuse within the family.[22] An overwhelming majority spoke about feeling neglected in the years of the pandemic.

From Mumbai's Andheri area came the poignant news of 'Uncle Joe', a seventy-five-year-old who had spent the last decade living in the basement of a housing society he was once the secretary of. He was thrown out by his family and had nowhere to go. He was found lying unconscious in the building's common washroom and was saved by the residents. Tests revealed that he was COVID positive and that he had also fractured his hip.

In Delhi, eighty-year-old Murlidhar Tahiliani posted a notice outside his house after running a fever for ten days and being suspected of having COVID. The poster said that should he die, his body must be handed over directly to the police.

Tahiliani, who had worked as an intelligence officer, had been abandoned by his family after they suspected he had COVID. It was left to a police constable, Raj Ram, to make sure that he got help at a hospital.

And from Krishna district came the horror story about the family that dialled a local NGO to ask for help in performing the last rites of an elderly woman who they said had died from COVID. But when local activists reached the apartment, they found that she was alive and had been placed under lock and key in her own house so she could not leave the premises. It was left to them to get her treated.

As soon as Leelawati's story was in the public domain there was a deluge of responses.

Everyone who saw what happened wanted to donate money, clothes and food.

Everyone wanted to know: What happened to that old lady stranded at the station in Bandra?

There were no trains running that evening and Leelawati had nowhere to go.

Senior officials of Western Railway made sure she did not spend the night out on the pavement, taking her inside to the safety and comfort of a waiting room. When she arrived in Delhi, she had changed her sari to a pale pink one. She was brought out in a wheelchair with a whole bunch of people attending to her. And she was beaming. 'I travelled in an air-conditioned coach and was given a lot of food to eat,' she declared happily.

By now, a man called Kiran Verma, whom I did not know, reached out to us from Delhi offering to take Leelawati in and legally adopt her. I was unsure of the best way to proceed and reached out to NGOs that work specifically with the elderly. Eventually, after much confabulation, everyone agreed that

Leelawati could spend a few days at Kiran's home and make up her own mind.

A few days later, Leelawati tested positive for COVID.

Kiran's family became anxious and were uneasy about having Leelawati become their responsibility. They felt she should be treated at a hospital.

Leelawati was in danger of being orphaned and homeless again when an entirely unlikely intervention was made by Sanjay Singh, parliamentarian with the Aam Aadmi Party. He made sure that she got proper medical attention and then took her home. 'She is like a family member,' he said later, as photographs of Leelawati sitting cross-legged on a diwan, flanked by Sanjay and his wife, went viral.

Of all her children, only her eldest daughter bothered to keep an eye Leelawati.

When I last checked on her, she had gone to spend some time with her daughter.

Leelawati was not an isolated case of an abandoned elderly citizen in India. There was something about Leelawati that broke your heart but also filled you with hope. In her tragedy – and then in her somewhat hopeful ending – perhaps we saw our worst and best selves.

In September 2020, as the worst of the first wave began winding down, Adar Poonawalla, the CEO of the Pune-based Serum Institute, was getting ready to send millions of vaccines into production. But the government did not place its formal order for vaccines till early January 2021. The failure to order enough vaccines early enough is probably the biggest mistake of the government's COVID response over two years. There was an odd mixture of denialism, complacency and misplaced exceptionalism, even at the highest levels of the administration. So, no one was prepared for Delta when it came. On 28 January 2021, PM Modi addressed the World Economic Forum in Davos and said that India has not just beaten COVID; it had helped 150 other countries. Two months later, in April, India was warring with the second avatar of the virus. By this time, caught in the stranglehold of the Delta variant, it was too late to use the vaccines as a way out of the storm.

With its massive experience in mass immunization, India's vaccine program eventually picked up impressive momentum and scale. By the first week of January 2022, India had administered 1.5 billion doses. Dramatic images of community health workers, crossing streams, climbing mountains, navigating thick forests and braving extreme temperatures to deliver the shots to the remotest areas made the country proud. But in some ways, these numbers and visuals also underscored what might have been achieved had more vaccines been ordered and rolled out earlier.

By the time the vaccine program found its rhythm, India had been brutalised by the second wave.

And just when it seemed as if India had slowly begun to heal from the wounds and gashes inflicted by Delta, the end of 2021 brought with it the arrival of Omicron. As this new variant readied to unleash a third wave on the country, a booster shot of the vaccine became imperative, even while India was still focused on inoculating its entire adult population with two jabs. On Christmas, the PM announced that the elderly and front-line workers would be prioritized for another shot of the vaccine. Despite the government's preference for a *swadeshi* vaccine that had been entirely developed and produced in India, multiple delays in trial data and WHO approval shadowed Covaxin, made by Bharat Biotech. And a persistent gap in its volume meant that by the end of 2021, the majority of those inoculated – 88 per cent – had been given Covishield, a vaccine developed at England's Oxford University and manufactured by the Poonawalla family.

6

'Nobody Teaches You this at Harvard'

A five-minute phone call from a son to his father is where it all began.

Adar Poonawalla was driving to work when he took the decision. His family's collection of luxury cars, including a custom-fitted Mercedes Batmobile, a Rolls-Royce and a Ferrari 458 Speciale Aperta, of which there are fewer than 500 units around the world, had always made it to the glossies. But today the flamboyant businessman's mind was elsewhere.

It was the month of April 2020 and a statement from the Jenner Institute at Oxford University announced a partnership with pharmaceutical giant AstraZeneca to develop a COVID vaccine.

Poonawalla knew Adrian Hill, the institute's director, because of their earlier collaboration on the malaria vaccine.

He felt the Serum Institute, the world's largest vaccine maker, could not sit this one out, despite the inherent risks. But he needed the approval of his father, Cyrus.

The Jenner Institute was named after Edward Jenner, the eighth of nine children born to a British vicar, and who was inoculated for smallpox as a child at school. The side effects would have a lifelong impact on Jenner's health. Eventually, he would be the scientist who would reimagine the modern smallpox vaccine by experimenting with cowpox, a mild viral infection in cows that did not appear to produce any major discomfort in humans. In the strange way that the dots of the universe sometimes conspire to connect, Jenner was awarded with the Degree of Doctor of Science, Honoris Causa, by the University of Oxford in 1813. More than 200 years later, in 2019, Cyrus Poonawalla became only the second person to be recognized with the same honorary doctorate. And a year later, his son was keen to work with the same institute to manufacture arguably the most important vaccine of the twenty-first century.

'Dad was apprehensive,' Adar said about his billionaire father, the son of a horse breeder with a love for Rembrandts, Brioni suits, thoroughbreds and a quintessentially Parsi joie de vivre, down to the discotheque built in the basement of his mansion. 'He has built things from scratch, so he always feels he has more to lose than I do,' Adar Poonawalla told me, with a laugh.

Cyrus Poonawalla, who got into the business of making vaccines after accidentally discovering that they used horse serum, was hardly regarded as fiscally conservative by the outside world. He partied with Paris Hilton, dined with Kate Middleton and posed unapologetically with his gulf streams. Risk was no stranger to his life. He and his brother Zavaray entered the vaccine manufacturing business with a 12-acre plot and a $12,000 investment, partially subsidized by their father. Yet, even by father Cyrus's zany standards, his son was taking an extraordinary, crazy risk.

Adar Poonawalla argued that it was in keeping with his ambition to expand capacity at the company. When he began work at Serum in 2001 at the age of twenty, their company exported vaccines to no more than forty nations. By the time Adar had turned thirty-six, they were present in 147 countries. It is estimated that about 65 per cent of children in the world receive at least one vaccine manufactured by the Serum Institute. In 2017, Adar, in constant pursuit of new technologies, declared that they would be able to launch a new vaccine in under a year and a half.

In 2020, that proclamation was put to the test like never before, with shorter timelines and without any agreed-on technology. Before COVID, the mumps vaccine was the fastest vaccine to be developed, taking four years.

'I won't stop you if you want to do it,' Cyrus said to Adar, 'but is it worth it to jump in like a mad man so early on?'

'This will be a race,' the son argued. 'If I can't be the first, I don't want to be the last,' Adar made his case.

'He has never stopped me, but he wasn't keen to take a chance like this,' Adar Poonawalla told me later, looking back at his audacity of those months.

Cyrus gave his consent but with a caveat. There was to be a finite budget – no more than $250 million of the company's resources were to be spent on the bungee jump into the deep end of science. At first, Adar thought it would be more than enough.

Now, they needed to find a contact at AstraZeneca to get an accelerated partnership status. There was no time for the normal round of Zoom calls and get-to-know negotiations. Time was of the essence, and though Adar declined to say yes or no, word is that Prince Charles helped expedite things. Charles had made a visit to the institute in Pune in 2013 and had asked sincere questions about measles and mumps. Adar and his wife Natasha also hosted Camilla and Charles for dinner at their 100-hectare farmhouse done up in metal and leather with a bespoke all-glass conservatory that opened up to a canopy of Australian pines.

A month later, the agreement with AstraZeneca was ready. The normally sluggish bureaucracy had also fast-tracked the ten licences needed for any vaccine to be made in India. And Poonawalla was set for what would be the biggest gamble of his professional life.

There was a reason he chose to back this particular vaccine, Poonawalla explained. 'I wanted to build a giant capacity. My choice was driven by yield,' he said, referring to the viral vector technology that powers the AstraZeneca, or the Covishield vaccine as we know it in India.

Traditional vaccines train your body to fight a pathogen by infecting you with a part of it. A vector-driven vaccine, by contrast, takes a harmless virus that delivers a genetic code to your cells that mimics the infective virus. The cells then make a protein that creates immunity. In other words, you acquire resistance without first being partially infected. The third category of COVID vaccines, the new and radical mRNA shots, relies on tricking your cells into making some of the viral proteins COVID would have normally produced, after which the cells mount a defence against them. While swifter to make to scale, they were not an option for Indian manufacturers because of the subzero storage requirements and demands for a complicated cold chain. And so, Serum Institute chose to throw its money and people behind a vaccine that used a chimpanzee common-cold virus to stimulate COVID immunity.

Even in peacetime, vaccine producers need a six-month head time to organize the raw material, glass vials, chemicals and plants required to bring out a vaccine. Now, as Adar and his team started doing the maths, they swiftly understood that to make the COVID vaccine they would have to stop or postpone the production of some other vaccine. Serum pushed back the launch of the HPV vaccine. The dengue monoclonal vaccine that had been announced in 2019 for unveiling within four years had to be paused. Plants that had been allocated for its production were taken over for the COVID vaccine.

But within a month of starting the process, Adar Poonawalla stopped sleeping at night. He would toss and turn as he did the numbers in his head and slipped into greater and greater panic. 'I had made a promise to the world,' Adar told me, 'and I was worried sick that I was going to fall short.'

He realized that the expenditure calculations he had made were way off the mark. As the COVID cases mounted, it was clear that he would need four times the $250 million cut-off the Institute had set. He considered approaching private banks and equity ventures for a loan or an investment. In the meantime, the company decided to sell a polio vaccine plant in Czechoslovakia to American pharmaceutical giant Novavax, raising $167 million from the deal. But they were still significantly short. 'You're getting in over your head,' Cyrus Poonawalla warned.

The Institute opened negotiations with a consortium of private equity firms – TPG Capital, Abu Dhabi's ADQ and Saudi Arabia's Public Investment Fund. But eventually it turned down an offer of $1 billion because of differences over valuation. A providential Zoom call with Bill Gates some time in May 2020 offered Adar a cushion to rest on. 'Are you willing to take a fifty-fifty risk,' Poonawalla asked Gates, underlining the urgent need to build high-volume capacity. Before the hour was up they had managed to shake hands on a deal. They agreed to price the vaccine at $3 per jab in low-income countries. Securing the promise that the Serum Institute would supply vaccines to emerging economies in Asia, Gates gave a thumbs-up to $300 million.

And Covishield went into mass production.

'I've never worked this hard in my life,' laughed Poonawalla, in an oblique acknowledgement of his enormous wealth and privilege. 'I would be up till 11 p.m. every night. I had to manage the expectations of the government, of governments in other countries, of the media, of people. I had to manage the risk I had taken. It was unheard of.'

By the end of September 2020, Serum had 600 million glass vials ready, made from special borosilicate glass that would protect the contents of the vaccine without chemically cross-wiring it. Winding down from the worst of the first outbreak at this time, the government had still not placed any advance requisitions with him. In other words, not a single vaccine had been ordered. Poonawalla set a target for himself anyway: 100 million doses per month would be available for India by the end of the year.

The phones were buzzing from other countries, though. Poonawalla hopped on to Zoom sessions with multiple heads of states, from Angela Merkel in Germany to Bolsonaro in Brazil; from countries in Africa to smaller nations nearer home, including Nepal and Bangladesh. Poonawalla created a differential pricing system and managed to lock in advance orders for $150 million with pre-delivery payments of 50 per cent.

Things between Poonawalla and the bureaucrats tasked with handling the COVID response as well as negotiating the price of vaccines began to get a little tense. 'It was a personality clash,' said one government official, describing the collision of mindsets between the plodding, conservative, slow-motion approach of a government system and the impatient, flamboyant, media-friendly CEO. While there is widespread acknowledgement that 'Serum is an excellent company', there is some obvious resentment at Poonawalla's ambitions. 'He wanted to run his own foreign policy,' said one government adviser, in a broadside at the direct hotlines Poonawalla had activated with prime ministers, presidents and health ministers across the globe. 'Why couldn't he just let his product speak for itself?'

However, Poonawalla knew that the global advance orders were critical to bridging the financial gap. Without that secured, the production pipelines would not work smoothly. There was already pressure on the infrastructure. Where he initially thought one vaccine plant, already installed with water and steam, would do, he now knew he needed at least five plants repurposed for COVID.

In India, the government gave its first order with the Serum Institue on 10 January 2021. Placed in context, these were not enough to provide the first dose to even the adult population of Delhi (150 million). To meet its own target for every Indian adult to be vaccinated by the end of 2021, the government needed to be administering these many shots every single day of the year. In March 2021, the national average for vaccination per million people stood at 11,675 doses. This number was 232,300 for the US and 314,100 for the UK.[23]

Admittedly comparisons between these nations are not straightforward. India's size, diversity, geography and terrain are entirely different. Still, history bears testimony to India's long experience with mass immunization as well as to a ready network of community workers who can accelerate the pace of vaccinations, even in the remotest interiors of the country, which is why the programme was able to pick up the kind of pace it did towards the latter half of 2021.

But in the winter of 2020 and the beginning of the new year, the vaccine programme was clearly thought of as incremental. Instead, the government was obsessed with the idea of a Made in India vaccine. That, and the calculation that vaccines could be used as an instrument of strategic soft power, made the government stumble on what was possibly the gravest of its mistakes in its COVID response. It simply failed to place a bulk order (or import) a substantial number of vaccines.

While this jousting went on behind closed doors for months through 2020, 150,000 people across 700 districts had been trained and readied to unveil the vaccine programme. Healthcare workers and doctors would be the first in line to get the shot. The roll-out was to begin on 16 January and the target was to vaccinate 300 million Indians by July. At this stage, India had already recorded the second highest number of infections in the world; the only country ahead was the US. But there was a sense of exceptionalism that had made India complacent. While the infections had been high in 2020, the relative mortality was significantly less compared to what obtained in the rest of the world. We had not yet confronted the phenomenon of mass undercounting of deaths – and in any case there was the belief that if people were dying unenumerated in the thousands, there would be a pile-up of bodies in hospital corridors or even on the streets again, as we would witness in the second wave. In the absence of any such visual triggers, in the beginning of the new year, India genuinely believed its trajectory had been different. And the data appeared to back the belief. In September 2020, as the crest of the first wave was beginning to plateau, Johns Hopkins reported how India's mortality rate – deaths for every 100 confirmed COVID cases – was 1.7 per cent, against 11.1 per cent in the UK and over 12 per cent in Italy. In September 2020, if India had 0.84 death per million, Brazil had 3.8 fatalities per million and the US 2.56 deaths per million. Early on in the first wave, Indian-American immunologist Siddhartha Mukherjee called the comparatively low death rates 'a mystery. To be frank I don't know and the world does not know why.'

In contrast to India's tardiness, the Americans had signed an agreement in July 2020 with Pfizer under Operation Warp Speed, so named after the Star Trek version of 'speed faster than light'. The agreement, signed before the phase-two trials, guaranteed 100 million doses of the Pfizer vaccine to the US with a provision for the US to acquire 1.3 billion vaccines by the end of 2021. It's a different matter that what ended up being warped was the American emphasis on personal liberty, so that even when vaccines were available aplenty, no mandates were ordered and nearly half the country opted not to take the jab. But the Biden administration signed a $1.9 billion agreement against an advance purchase for a vaccine that had not yet cleared trials.

In India, only 2 per cent of the adult population had been vaccinated by May when the number of cases peaked at 400,000 per day.

Within the government, the blame was placed at the door of the affable but bumbling Health Minister Harsh Vardhan and the bureaucrat-in-chief of the time, Vinod Paul.

'The biggest mistake we made was to not bulk-order vaccines in the autumn of 2020,' said a top official. 'It was bureaucratic inertia. It was also because not a single bureaucrat was ready to put his name to an order that paid money in advance. It was just not in their way of thinking.'

With no purchase order from within India, Poonawalla began exporting vaccines to the countries that had agreed to pay upfront, covering more than sixty nations. 'I was planting the flag of Indian pharmacy on the global stage,' he told me.

His proclamation that ₹80,000 crore (around $10 billion) would need to be budgeted for India's COVID response had irritated the government. In a sharp rebuff, the health secretary dismissed the numbers. 'We do not agree with the calculation. The government has made a national committee of vaccine experts and five meetings have taken place. We have mulled over the process of vaccine distribution and the amount required for it in terms of prioritization of population and the staggered immunization for this prioritization.'

The formal structure of the language, the choice of words – 'mulled over', 'staggered' – said everything about the slow-moving manner in which the administration approached the question of vaccines.

Poonawalla's estimates were based on his assumption that the vaccines in India would be priced at $4 per shot and that universal vaccination of a billion people over two years would cost India $8 billion, which translated into roughly ₹60,000 crore. He thought India would also purchase some vaccines from Pfizer and Moderna, which had priced their shots at $7 each. And another $2.68 billion (₹20,000 crore) would need to be ploughed into managing the hospital system and building a cold chain. The mRNA vaccines could only be stored at temperatures below 2 degrees Celsius, and Poonawalla believed the government would purchase at least a percentage of the Institute's vaccines since they were first off the block and already available.

But entangled in a disagreement over who would provide legal cover – Pfizer and Moderna wanted the same indemnity they had from other governments across the world – and fixated on the idea of a 'Made in India' vaccine, India never went down that route.

Instead, Krishna Ella, a study in contrast to the glamorous Poonawalla, was tasked with the development of Covaxin, a traditional vaccine that used killed (inactivated) coronaviruses to prompt the immune system. Ella, born to a family of farmers in a village in Tamil Nadu, had studied in the US on a Rotary scholarship and had returned to set up Bharat Biotech with his wife Suchitra, with seed funding of ₹12 crore ($1.61 million), borrowed from savings and bank loans. Though Bharat Biotech sells vaccines in seventy countries, Covaxin was mired in controversy from its inception. The government's decision to give it emergency-use authorization before its phase-three trials were completed creating conspiratorial doubts about its efficacy. For the first three months of the vaccine roll-out, this meant that you had to sign a consent form if you were going to be jabbed with Covaxin. It was not until November 2021 that it received approval from the WHO.

Poonawalla even took a swipe at the homespun vaccine by saying that it was 'safe like water'. Ella fumed back. The government had to step in to get the two to make up and issue a tetchy joint statement.

It wasn't till the prime minister got his shot – and underlined that it was the India-developed one – that the narrative turned. In fact, this time it swung the other way, with whispers about Covaxin being the safer shot to take. In much the same way the government-run public sector units were once considered safer than the imagined ad hocism of the profit-fixated private sector, influential people connected to government, who could choose where they could get vaccinated and which vaccine they could get, opted for Covaxin over Covishield.

That honeymoon didn't last long. Ella, described by one government official as 'an eccentric scientist without business acumen or production capacity', may have been pushed far too hard by the government to be the poster child for its homespun vaccine. Not just were health experts troubled by the initial lack of transparency around the data on Covaxin, but even when the vaccine was proved to be effective at a nearly 80 per cent rate against the coronavirus, Bharat Biotech repeatedly fell short of its production targets. Nine months after its approval, by September 2021, only one in every eleven Indians was getting injected with Covaxin because of the constant shortfall in predicted supplies. The government amended its own response in the Supreme Court, modifying the 100 million doses it had initially claimed would come from Covaxin to 80 million. But when questions were raised in Parliament, the government offered a dramatically lower figure, one that changed three times in a single month, ranging from 10 million to 20 million shots a month. Essentially, Ella's company was producing less than half of what it had promised.

Poonawalla and Ella may have sniped in public, but the one time they were on the same side was during negotiations over what their vaccines should be priced at. 'They were ugly negotiations and went on for a month,' said a representative of the vaccine industry who was present in the room. Pfizer had priced itself at $20 with the Biden administration; Indian vaccine manufacturers felt they should be allowed to price the dose at at least ₹500 per shot. Eventually, the first 100 million doses purchased by the government in January were priced at ₹200 each and paid for by the PM Cares Fund, an emergency-care corpus that had been set up in response to COVID in 2020. Thereafter, once private hospitals were allowed to administer vaccines, the government initially capped the price at ₹250 a shot, of which ₹100 covered hospital service costs and the remaining ₹150 went to the vaccine makers.

Manufacturers were agitated and furious in the closed-door meetings with V.K. Paul and a team of bureaucrats.

At one stage, Poonawalla in particular got so exasperated he considered terminating the agreement to produce vaccines. He told the government negotiators that the pricing was so absurd that COVID tests cost twice as much as the vaccine, and in some states three and four times higher. 'You are destroying our industry,' he told impassive bureaucrats who attended the negotiations, representing multiple ministries of pharmaceuticals, health and biotech. He argued that a reasonable margin of profit was essential to build capacity – plants, personnel, skilled scientists – for exactly such a crisis as COVID. The government was unmoved.

Poonawalla worried that he would be caricatured as a profit seeker in the middle of a crisis. Steel tycoon Sajjan Jindal publicly criticized Poonawalla in comments to the *Financial Times* urging him to drop his price and 'work with the government'. His friends say Poonawalla was hurt and angry. 'Do you want me to be a mahatma,' he retorted in private. 'I do not have a magic wand.'

Eventually the government had its way. 'We do not have the budget,' declared V.K. Paul with the firmness of an auctioneer bringing down the hammer on the final price. 'And Mr Poonawalla, you are very efficient, I am sure you will manage.'

And so, three days after the vaccines were unveiled and prioritized for health workers and doctors in the first phase, the foreign ministry announced its decision to 'use India's vaccine production and capacity to help all of humanity fight the covid pandemic'.

Unaware of the crisis that lay ahead, most Indians, including myself, welcomed the government's move. There was something uplifting about seeing Indian Air Force plane loads take off with vaccines manufactured in India. It was only when the shortage of vaccines was revealed right in the middle of the second wave that what the government had been praised for started looking like an egotistical and ill-conceived decision. People demanded to know why Indians had not been prioritized first. Under the Vaccine Maitri scheme, 94.5 million doses had been dispatched for use in ninety-six countries. But if you break down the data, you see that only 12.7 million of these had been sent as grants by the government. The remaining 54.7 million vaccine doses were actually part of the commercial obligations that the Serum Institute made in its agreement with AstraZeneca. A bureaucrat remarked laconically that the government was riding on Poonawalla's back as it made India seem expansive, generous and responsible. Till, of course, the second wave stormed through the heart of the country and what had looked benevolent suddenly looked bizarre. Vaccine exports remained banned from April to September of 2021.

In the end, Poonawalla was vindicated despite all the carping. Eighty-eight per cent of India was inoculated with vaccines made at the Serum Institute. AstraZeneca was the most widely administered vaccine in the world.

'I have learnt how to deal with crises now. Perhaps I was a bit green earlier. Nobody taught me how to deal with such a public situation. We have always been a private company. Nobody teaches this at Harvard and Stanford,' Adar Poonawalla told me. 'I don't have any regrets. Looking back, I wouldn't have done anything differently. Perhaps I could have stayed a little more silent. But I felt certain issues had to be responded to. Because sometimes there was so much noise and a lack of communication. It could have been better from all parties; we could have all explained things to the people of India better.'

But 2021 ended with an ironic déjà vu. With the spectre of a new variant, Omicron, haunting the world, consensus built up globally on the need for a third or booster shot. Though scientists advocated for an mRNA jab to be the booster, in the absence of these vaccines in India it was argued that at least the elderly and health workers should be boosted with Covishield. Even with reduced effectiveness, a third jab was considerably more protection against serious disease than no jab at all. Poonawalla told me that the demand had fallen by almost 80 per cent. He dashed off letters to officials in the government asking for 'guidance' on what to do with the stockpile of 200 million vaccines ready in the pipeline. He was running out of storage capacity and offered to send the reserve stocks to government storage depots.

2021 ended the same way as 2020 in one respect: there were no government orders for vaccines in the coming year, at least not up until 24 December 2021.

'But I am ready,' said Poonawalla, 'now I have learnt,' talking about his capacity to turn things around even at short notice.

On Christmas evening, the prime minister addressed the nation. Booster shots, he said, would begin from the first week of January for health workers and the elderly.

When the second wave arrived in India in March 2021, the first response to it was denial; the second was defiance. Public events – election rallies and mass congregations – continued till 22 April when the prime minister decided to suspend his physical campaign in West Bengal, falling back on remotely conducted virtual speeches instead. Controversially, neither the courts nor the Election Commission stepped in to stop the polling process and the crowd-gathering it encouraged. Among the first victims of this misplaced and irresponsible focus on electoral politics in the middle of a pandemic were the government school teachers of Uttar Pradesh. They were forced to attend poll duty for local elections on the insistence of the Allahabad High Court, leading to mass COVID deaths within a fraternity that was never given the right to choose.

7

'They Have Blood on Their Hands'

Jaunpur, in the eastern corner of Uttar Pradesh, has long been used to living in the shadows of adjacent Varanasi, grander for its civilizational history and religious significance, as well for as its primacy in the political pecking order as Prime Minister Narendra Modi's Parliament seat. In the past two years of COVID, residents of Jaunpur have often travelled the 60-kilometre distance to their more developed neighbour in search of better hospitals and even cremation grounds.

The wilting grandeur of the city, once conquered by the Mughal emperor Akbar in 1559, is best captured by its Shahi Pul, a unique stone bridge over the Gomti river, punctuated by symmetrically separated pillboxes, from which, once upon a time, traders sold their wares. On a square platform in the middle of the bridge is a sculpture of a giant lion lumbering over an elephant, apparently to illustrate the vanquishing of Buddhism in the sixteenth century.

In 2021, every time Deepak Agrahari rides past it on his Super Splendour motorcycle, pushed around by the paperwork demands of one government office after another, it feels a lot like his own life, one crushed under the gigantic and intimidating weight of a hostile, non-compassionate state. Like the elephant, Deepak has been vanquished.

The only time he smiles is when he shares the photographs of his wife Kalyani – in red silk draping her bejewelled frame on the day they got married, in an emerald green sari she wore with a contrasting black blouse when they went on vacation, wearing the mangalsutra she never took off, sporting a river of red sindoor running through the expanse of her thick black hair and, occupying pride of place in his phone album, a photograph of the school where she would soon be teaching.

It was on 27 January that Kalyani was appointed to her dream job as assistant teacher at Composite Vidyalaya, Khuthan, an English-medium school in the rural outback of Jaunpur, roughly 30 kilometres from the spot where the lion towered over the elephant.

All her life Kalyani had wanted to be a teacher and she could scarcely believe that it was all finally falling into place. In fact, personally and professionally, Kalyani had never been happier. Married to Deepak in April 2018, she was less than two months away from giving birth to their first child. It also made her heart fill with pride that for the next few months she was going to be the main earning member of their household. Deepak had quit his low-paying job in a boiler factory nearly 700 kilometres away; he wanted to be closer to his wife and baby. Kalyani's government job would earn just over ₹30,000 a month and Deepak, who had a bachelor's degree in technology (BTech), would use the time to find work closer home.

But before schools could reopen and she could step into a classroom, Kalyani was summoned for election duty. Panchayat elections, touted as an all-important prelude to the high-voltage battle for Uttar Pradesh in 2022, were going to be held on 15 April 2021; government teachers had long been deployed at election centres to oversee the voting process in the country.

Despite being eight months pregnant, Kalyani was hesitant to appear fussy. What if it cost her the first job she'd ever had. Deepak would hear none of it. The dangers of COVID aside, the pregnancy was at too precarious a stage for her to take a risk. They decided to write and ask for exemption from the district officials deputed to conduct the polls, citing a 'critical pregnancy' and the inherent dangers. No one replied.

On the eve of the elections, Deepak accompanied his wife to the polling booth at the Karanjakala block. They thought they would make a last-minute effort to convince the administration to excuse Kalyani from election duty. Then they heard the warnings being made on loudspeaker. 'Anyone who fails to show up will face disciplinary action.'

Of all the egregious mistakes and acts of negligence by India's institutions, none comes close to the decision to hold multi-phase elections to both state assemblies and local bodies right through the second wave of COVID. Polls equalled gigantic crowds in the thousands, pushing and jostling for space, perilously proximate during a pandemic where every single expert had warned that 'even two people were a crowd'.

On 17 April, the Union health minister, Harsh Vardhan, admitted to 'a sharp growth of 10 per cent' in COVID deaths, warning that 'new cases are rising alarmingly'. That week the country had officially recorded 200,000 cases every day for three consecutive days.

On the same day, Asansol – where the sooty coal mines have almost denuded the asan tree after which West Bengal's second largest city is named – had a visitor. His candyfloss beard had now grown out in cascades of white but his pitch-perfect performer's voice still had the same mastery over the stage aside whisper. Prime Minister Modi was sans a mask but he wore his best Amitabh Bachchan voice as he shared his faux hurt with the mammoth crowd. His 'bittersweet complaint' was that when he had come previously during the national elections to campaign for himself, 'one-fourth the number of people had shown up. And now, *jahan dekhta hoon, log hi log dikhte hai.*' (Wherever I look, for as far as the eye can see, I see people.) The crowd roared in approval.

In the next twenty-four hours India's official deaths from COVID climbed to 1,500 and daily new cases breached the 260,000 mark.

The prime minister's brag about large numbers at his rally, at a time when localized lockdowns were pushing citizens indoors in most of non-election-bound India, was dangerously mixed messaging. It was the exhortation of mass congregation in one part of India and the urging of 'COVID-appropriate behaviour' in others. And it's not as if gentle persuasion was being used elsewhere to keep people from stepping out of their homes. While not as draconian as the all-India curfew template of 2020, restrictions on movement of people were still police enforced. At mustard-yellow traffic barricades in all major cities where elections weren't being held, police waved down cars and scooters to check who was out for what reason, mostly slowing down the free movement of ambulances in the process.

On 27 February, when the Election Commission announced the schedule for the five states (Kerala, Assam, Tamil Nadu, West Bengal and Puducherry) where new assemblies were being voted in, India was already adding close to 17,000 new cases every day. Eighty-five per cent of new cases were from six states, of which one was Kerala. Yet, voting for Kerala was scheduled for 6 April, allowing for one month of crowds, rallies and risky exposure. In Assam, on the campaign trail, Himanta Biswa, the flamboyant BJP minister seen to be the party's key strategist, justified his not wearing a mask by declaring that 'there is no corona' in the eastern state. In the two-month period of April and May, twice as many people died from COVID than they had all year in 2020. West Bengal had the longest election spread over eight phases, finishing only by the end of April.

On the day that the prime minister was in Asansol, 1,341 Indians had died from COVID in the previous 24 hours.

Three days before his giant rally, Shahid Jameel, pre-eminent virologist, warned: 'I think we have lost the plot. Just wait to see what comes out of Bengal. What I see happening today, you will see the implications of it in a month. You cannot have mass gatherings where millions gather and not call them super-spreader events. There will be mutant strains that may evade vaccines.'

It wasn't the BJP alone that was conducting itself imprudently. Political parties across the spectrum were complicit with their very participation in these elections instead of taking a unanimous call to postpone them.

On 1 May – by this time oxygen, beds and drugs were running out at hospitals that were shutting their doors to critically ill patients – Chief Justice Sanjib Banerjee at the Madras High Court tore into the institution that had blood on its hands – the Election Commission. Banerjee, whose home state is West Bengal and who once covered cricket and tennis as a sports journalist for the *Telegraph* newspaper before becoming a lawyer, lashed out at the constitutional body for its business-as-usual attitude. 'You are singularly responsible for the second wave. You should be tried for murder. Were you on another planet when election rallies were held?' By now India's (official) daily deaths had climbed to 3,673.

Banerjee seemed to be among the handful of Indians of consequence who had paid close attention to warnings of a second wave in October 2020. Then, still a judge in the Calcutta High Court, he decreed that Durga Puja pandals be cordoned off and treated as no-entry zones. No more than fifteen to twenty members of organizing committees in every pandal would be permitted to gather at the 37,000 pandals across the state. They would have to be treated as containment zones under the court's orders.

Five months later, in stark contrast to these restrictions, starting in the second week of March, hundreds of thousands of pilgrims were permitted to gather by the banks of the Ganga at the Kumbh Mela in Haridwar, in the state of Uttarakhand. A religious festival held four times every twelve years and organized in accordance with planetary positions, the Kumbh travels to sites on four rivers regarded as holy by Hindus – the Ganga, the Shipra, the Godavari and the Sangam (confluence) in Prayagraj.

In April alone, while places of worship elsewhere in India, especially gurudwaras, rushed to organize oxygen 'langars' so that those who could not get an oxygenated hospital bed might at least get temporary respite from a cylinder made available to them for a handful of minutes, upwards of 6 million Indians arrived for the 'Shahi Snan' or holy bath in Haridwar. That a Persian word captures the centrepiece of a Hindu ritual is noteworthy because it's a throwback to the messy, shared, sometimes overlapping cultural history of the Indian people. The other noteworthy point was how markedly different the response had been a year earlier to a much smaller congregation of the Tablighi Jamaat, an orthodox Muslim sect, in Delhi. In

2020, many news channels had used the skullcap as the visual backdrop for statistical representation of COVID cases in clear communal signalling. A poisonous anti-Muslim rhetoric was actively incited. This time, the condemnation of the Haridwar event was muted, even perfunctory. The chief minister of Uttarakhand, the blundering, bumbling Tirath Singh Rawat, known for his headline-seeking inanities, rejected any analogy of the Kumbh with the Jamaat. Even as 2,000 pilgrims tested positive for COVID within five days of their arriving for the event, Rawat insisted that the 'flow and blessings of Ma Ganga' would insulate devotees from the virus.

It was only on 17 April – yes, the same day that the prime minister applauded the gigantic crowds in West Bengal – that he also 'requested' the seers of the Kumbh to keep the remaining days 'symbolic'. And he physically withdrew himself from campaigning five days later, when just the last phase of the election was left.

All the giant gatherings – the state election rallies, the Kumbh, the funeral processions and weddings, and even the farmers from Punjab and Haryana who soldiered on with protests at the borders of the capital – were rooted in different impulses. But each such event had the consent of its participants.

The only set of people literally consigned to death by the Indian State were the government teachers of Uttar Pradesh, who were forcibly deployed on election duty. They were robbed of all agency to make a choice for themselves. Those who tried to push back were threatened with being sacked. Or worse, with criminal cases. The Indian State that had gone absent for the vast majority of its people in containing COVID was instinctively overweening and intimidating in forcing thousands of men and women into elections that should never have been held at all.

By the middle of May, over 1,600 teachers in UP had died after exposure to the virus from either training workshops ahead of the voting or from being stationed at booths where crowds mingled and milled about, and which were visited by hordes of people pushing and pressing against each other. The teachers' unions would compile every death, neatly arranging their collective tragedy into columns, sheets and numbers, in the hope that the compilation would be treated as evidence of their having died from COVID picked up during election duty. They would send letter upon letter to the Yogi Adityanath government and to the national media. But for the most part, the deaths that actually amounted to culpable homicide barely triggered any outrage.

In homes across the dusty districts of India's most populous and politically important state, entire families were wiped out. At the north-eastern edge of the state, right on the border with Nepal, in Siddharthnagar, named after the Buddha's childhood name, Aniket pulled out a photograph of his parents, Lallan Ram and Meena Kumari, wide smiles on their faces as they posed shoulder to shoulder against a string of glittering coloured lights. The shiny bulbs formed a small halo over his father's shining bald pate, while his mother, with spectacles firmly on her nose, had the self-assurance of an economically independent professional woman. Meena ensured that Aniket's sister, Preeti, would have the same education as her brother. Preeti followed her parents' path and also became a teacher.

Preeti's sorrow is tinged with rage. 'They have murdered my parents, they have orphaned us when our schools were shut and our classrooms closed. What was the need to hold this election at all? At least they could have spared the elderly, the aged among us teachers, like my parents.'

Preeti started running a high fever three days after being posted on election duty in Gorakhpur, the erstwhile parliamentary constituency of the UP chief minister who goes by the prefix of 'Yogi' from his years as the chief priest of the Gorakhpur Math. In 2002, the saffron-robed rabble-rouser, who that year had launched a militant youth movement called 'Hindu Vahini', establishing a Hindutva hegemony independent of the BJP or the Rashtriya Swayamsevak Sangh (RSS).

His government has blamed the Allahabad High Court for insisting that the local elections not be delayed. The administration argues that it was forced into the scheduled elections on court orders.

Families who lost their loved ones blame all three institutions – the Election Commission, the high court and the Adityanath government.

The brute enforcement of government diktats, official and unofficial – this is a state where purported 'anti-Romeo squads' spread terror by often invading the privacy of consenting adults – made defying an official order almost impossible.

That day the enormity of grief had given that suppressed rage courage to express itself. '*Mein cheekh cheekh ke kahoongi*, the government murdered my parents,' Preeti said, her voice falling to an ironic whisper. 'I hold the state government responsible for orphaning us and murdering our parents. And I am ready to shout it from the rooftops.'

Applications were made, doctors' certificates were submitted, letters were written, hands were folded in submission . . . but no mercy was granted to families who sought exemption from election duty.

The teachers were literally summoned to their death. And then were made to pay for it.

Like hundreds of thousands of other Indians, their families struggled to find them beds, and if they were lucky enough to get a hospital admission they had to dip into their retirement savings or borrow from banks and local moneylenders to pay the bills.

By the time Lallan Ram was able to get admitted to a Gorakhpur hospital – his son had to beg a bureaucrat for help – doctors said it was already too late.

As his father lay in the ICU in the final days of his life, Aniket received a call from a government official inquiring about why his father was missing from poll duty. When Aniket explained that his father was running a COVID fever and they had already placed a formal application for leave, the officer snarled back, 'We will have to file an FIR [First Information Report], you can explain your response then.' Aniket cremated his father and returned home to find his mother Meena had also contracted the infection.

Ten days later, Meena passed on at Gorakhpur's district hospital. The family saw four other bodies in the same ward Meena died in. 'There were people who died in the bathroom, unattended, forgotten, they were just lying on the floor,' said Aniket. 'The staff did not even look at them.' Aniket and Preeti fought with the hospital authorities and demanded answers. 'Yogi Baba should come here and see what is happening, nothing that he promises actually translates on the ground. This is the chief minister's constituency. Surely the hospitals here should be better.'

What followed was social ostracism by the neighbourhood. 'No one has come to even condole,' said Preeti, stoic like her mother. 'Now that we are all alone we just have to find some way to pass the days. *Hamare paas koi shabd nahin bache.* (We have no words left.) My parents are gone, but for those who are alive can we at least have better facilities in our hospitals?'

Preeti regretted having become a teacher. 'Maybe if my parents had not chosen to be educationists, they would be alive today. At least we would have been more than mere numbers.'

In every such home children have been forced into early adulthood. They have become the consolers and comfort-givers to broken parents, elder siblings. They are often the only reason for those who may have lost the will to live to keep going. Three hundred kilometres from Siddharthnagar, in the city of Sitapur, a fifteen-year-old school student put an arm around her mother, Savita Devi, and urged her not to cry. 'My husband is number sixty-six on that list.' Savita, also a government teacher, was inconsolable talking about her husband Abhishek. '*Hum barbaad ho gaye, hamara sab kuch lut gaya.* (We are ruined. We have nothing left.) I have a four-year-old child, elderly parents: how will I look after them?'

Her teenage daughter wanted to share notes on grief with me. 'I heard your father died too,' said Vashvi Shukla, pushing her too-big-for-her-eyes glasses up the bridge of her nose, her big black eyes staring at me from behind them. 'You know how I feel then. When your father goes, you feel the person who will keep you secure and safe is gone. That's how I feel.'

Vashvi spoke without rancour and she spoke softly. But her words were unforgiving. 'I think the government does not have any respect for teachers. Nor do they have any value for human life. We all know this could have been avoided. Everything can be done online in today's world. They just wanted to play their dirty politics. I am traumatized. I have lost my father at such a young age. They have played with the lives of millions of people. I want to ask Adityanath, what was the need to do this. When even the Centre and the state governments are unable to fulfil their responsibilities towards the people during this pandemic, what have we achieved by holding elections to local bodies? What was the need for this?'

The daughter's eyes held no tears. Her mother, who was sitting by her side, was unable to hold them back. Every few minutes Vashvi reached for Savita's hand and held it tightly, giving her the strength to complete her sentences through a blizzard of tears. Abhishek was not able to survive more than two days in the district hospital. When Savita took him to be admitted the doctors were not prepared to even examine him. They had no PPE kits, not even a pair of gloves. Savita handed a doctor a pair of shiny blue plastic gloves she'd worn and persuaded him to take her husband in. 'They had oxygen but nothing else – no staff, no drugs, nothing. I touched the doctor's feet and begged him to at least place Abhishek on a drip. It took me three hours to convince them. For every injection I would touch their feet. Ward boys are running the hospital. They had no personnel at all.'

When her father died, it was left to Vashvi to run around and get the entire family tested for COVID. 'Even on that day, when they knew my father had died, not one person in the local administration was willing to help us. I try and be strong for my mother but some days it gets too tough.'

Neither Savita nor Vashvi believe there is any hope of justice. 'If the Centre or the state government wanted, they could have stopped this. They had both the power and the understanding of what this could do in the middle of the pandemic,' said the teenager.

There is the rare teacher's family that also sees signs of noble sacrifice and public service in the COVID deaths of their own. One of them is Satyadev Tiwari's. His brother Ashwini was in his forties and a father of two young girls. Like everyone else, Ashwini believed that if he did not show up for duty he could get a government notice or even an arrest warrant. By the time Satyadev was able to move him to a larger hospital in Gorakhpur, 70 per cent of Ashwini's lungs were already damaged and it was too late to save him. The trauma of losing his son was too much for their father, who died from a heart attack exactly a week later.

'We have been abandoned. No one from the administration has come to even look us up,' said Satyadev, who lives in a small one-room tenement with his aged mother.

In this family there is no trace of anger. Instead, there is just a sorrowful acceptance of an individual citizen's powerlessness to do anything when the state decides otherwise. 'My son could not violate government orders,' said Ashwini's mother. 'I am not an educated woman. But I know that my son did his duty. I am proud I gave birth to such a boy. Like my boy there are thousands of other such boys. They also have grieving mothers. My *shraddhanjali* to all of them.'

Ashwini's family try to console themselves by believing his life was lost in the line of duty. 'This was for democracy,' said his mother, when in fact the very holding of elections during the pandemic and not allowing thousands of teachers, whose core job had nothing to do with the electoral process, any say in their own lives, was the exact opposite: a shameful subversion of the democratic process.

As of June 2021, Adityanath's government had acknowledged the death of only three government teachers from COVID.

'They all have blood on their hands,' said Deepak, whose wife Kalyani died on 24 April, two days before their second wedding anniversary, along with their still-to-be-born baby.

Everything ran short in the peak months of the second wave – vaccines, oxygen, hospital beds, ambulances and drugs. Despair gave birth to a community of grief as people turned to each other for help. Civil society had to supplement – and in many cases substitute for – institutional responses to COVID as the system crumbled under the weight of Delta. Twitter became a message board for notices about plasma, remdesivir and oxygen concentrators. The kindness of strangers saw many people through the worst months of their lives. I was away in Maharashtra when I got the phone call I had dreaded all these months. What unfolded next made me the very story I had been reporting.

8

Fathers and Daughters

They say it gets better with time.

But it doesn't really.

The first thing that has altered in my life is that I cannot listen to music any more.

My father, S.P. Dutt, Speedy Dutt to friends and family alike, used to spend hours at his ramshackle workstation, sitting in a corner of his airless room amid a mountain of books, dusty files and meccano toys that he had designed and built, listening to music on internet radio stations.

Christmas carols, soft rock, Santana – there was a 24/7 loop of music on his ageing Apple desktop.

Every time I hear the opening chords of a song, a memory draws me back to that image of him and I feel the pain cut me like a knife.

It seems easier to not listen to any music at all.

I had begun to think of myself as peculiar till I read an account by Michelle Zauner in the *New Yorker* about how she would collapse in tears every time she went to shop at H-Mart, the Korean supermarket chain; the dry food cans triggered an immediate association with her mother.

Memory can be a beast.

That is my abiding personal lesson from the pandemic.

Before his death, my sister Bahar and I always valorized our mother, Prabha Dutt, whom we lost when I was just thirteen years old to a brain haemorrhage. She was a flamboyant, volatile, tempestuous counterfoil to the gentle, unassuming, kindly and eccentric man her husband was. Among the first generation of women journalists in India, she was the automatic headline story of our family. Notoriously rebellious, she was India's first woman war correspondent, reporting from the front line of the India-Pakistan war in 1965 by herself, armed with only a notepad and pen. We grew up in her shadow, moulded by extraordinary stories of how she once jumped into a hippopotamus enclosure to chase a story, how she petitioned the court and entered the annals of Indian case law by insisting on interviewing child murderers Billa and Ranga before they were executed, and how she exposed corruption and wrongdoing through her writings in the *Hindustan Times*. She was a legend, and because she died so young – she was just forty – the memory of her grew larger than life in our heads.

It was easy to take the person right in front of us – our dad – for granted.

It took losing him to COVID for me to realize how he had been the epicentre of my existence.

It took his death for me to understand how traumatized he must have been, especially as a single parent, every time I left for an assignment to a dangerous hotspot. I remember his protestations and anxieties two decades ago when I was dispatched to report on the Kargil war in 1999; I was dismissive, impatient and stubborn. And the truth is, he set me free, entirely so, even when he had to sit on his hands.

Every day I curse myself for not appreciating him as fully as I should have when he was alive.

And now it is too late.

I have lost count of the number of daughters I have met in my travels across India who are similarly haunted. By loss. By regret. By anger. By what-ifs.

And by memory.

In April 2021, during the peak of the second wave, one of Mumbai's most popular radio jockeys, Samridhi Saxena, better known as RJ Sam, desperately reached out to me in the hope that I could help her father with an oxygen cylinder. He had tested positive for COVID in 2020 and survived. Now he was struggling with a rare neurodegenerative disease and was on assisted breathing. Oxygen was as critical to keep him alive as it was for someone whose respiratory system was hit badly by the virus. Sam was ready to beg, borrow and steal, and did everything she could. She went on to Twitter, called everyone she knew, cried in front of strangers, folded hands in humility, snapped in exasperation. 'If someone is a non-COVID patient, doesn't he have the right to live? Doesn't he have the right to medical facilities?' Sam had created an ICU at home for her father, renting specialized equipment at the cost of ₹100,000 a month. But she could not get a single oxygen station in Mumbai to refill his now-depleted cylinders. 'I don't think he will survive,' she said, breaking down. A cylinder that normally cost ₹5,000 before the second wave had escalated to ₹9,000 in February 2021, and during the peak of the surge was as much as ₹45,000 in the black market.[24]

Betrayed by the state and the system, citizens formed a

community of their own for support during the worst months of the second wave. As we travelled through India, we were approached often by complete strangers who would track us down on social media or hunt down our number and cold-call us, in the desperate hope that we could do something that doctors had been unable to.

Usually, we were even more helpless than they were.

All I could do was listen, share their pain and tell their stories.

From Patna, another heartbroken daughter, Manisha, called me to say her fifty-three-year-old father would die because Ford Hospital, where both he and his wife were admitted for COVID, was asking the family to move him. 'He is critical, his oxygen is falling.' Manisha spoke breathlessly, as if her own heart would come to a crashing halt any moment. Like so many hospitals across India, this one too was dealing with a depleting supply in its ICU. Its administration advised that Manisha should either go out and organize the oxygen or find another medical facility. 'My father sent me a text message yesterday,' Manisha told me, 'since then I have heard nothing.' She knew the worst was imminent.

In Bengaluru I met twenty-one-year-old Bharini who asked me a question I had no answer to. 'How strong am I expected to be?' We were in her kitchen, seated on the ledge talking. I was still trying to wrap my head around her extraordinary tragedy. She lost her biological parents when she was very young and was adopted by her mother's sister and her husband. In 2021, she lost her adoptive father to a heart attack; later in the year her mother died from COVID. Though Bharini dreamt of being an IAS officer, on the day I met her she described herself as someone who was 'emotionally, mentally and financially broken'.

I was speechless. My own pain seemed unworthy compared to the magnitude of what she was struggling with.

But then, as Joan Didion, who also died in 2021, had first taught us, 'A single person is missing for you and the whole world is empty.'

Journalist Stutee Ghosh and I shared the sense of dissonance that came from remaining functional while you have a parent locked away in hospital, whom you have no access to. We spoke of the callousness of a glitzy IPL cricket tournament, a cash-rich advertising property, running right through the crisis, suspended only when players started testing positive despite their 'bio-bubble'. And we mirrored each other's persistent, gnawing guilt – that somehow we were letting down our fathers; and guilty also that even in the worst moment of our lives we were distinctly better off than hundreds of thousands of other Indians, just by the fact that our dads were in hospital, and we outside the closed gates of one. 'For the past nine days, I wake up with my phone and I go to sleep with my phone and when I am not calling someone for my father, I am, like everyone else, receiving or sending SOS messages for others, for an oxygen cylinder, or a bed, or medicine, or a concentrator, or warm food. I don't even know where the IPL is being played,' said Stutee. Her father, like mine, didn't make it. And, over the weeks, her grief mutated, like the virus, into rage at 'the indignity in death for so many Indians who are dying and not even being counted by the government.'

We were bereft. As daughters. And as citizens.

In April 2021, when the news first came from Delhi that my father had tested positive for COVID, I was on the road chasing the virus in Maharashtra, which at that point had the highest number of cases. I was sitting on the pavement outside the crematorium in Ghatkopar in Mumbai, fighting back tears as an elderly man in his nineties sat stoically in a wheelchair, waving a silent goodbye to his wife.

Initially, my father's infection seemed mild, and though he was in his eighties and a long-time patient of diabetes, the doctors thought it was easily manageable at home. That evening, on my digital platforms, I wrote about needing to find the balance between being a distraught daughter and a clear-headed, committed professional. I carried on reporting, travelling through the smaller towns of Maharashtra and onwards to Gujarat, where in Surat there were so many people dying every day that two iron furnaces at one of the city's biggest crematoriums had melted and corroded because too many corpses had been lit on them.

But when my father's fever persisted, I cut short my reporting assignment and flew back, a process that came with its own delays, because I first needed an all-clear on a COVID test.

I went to see him in the home where I had lived with him pretty much all my life up until the age of forty. My father's family, that once lived in a giant kothi with pillars made of white marble, dozens of rooms, fountains out in the infinite green lawns and a grand piano in its chandeliered living room, left Sialkot in pre-Partition Punjab and arrived in Delhi as penniless refugees. The capital took in half a million refugees before August 1947. My grandfather, Krishan Gopal Dutt, imprisoned during the freedom movement, died before I was born. His sons were allotted a small plot in colonies (like Jangpura Extension, where we stayed) that were created for such migrants near and around Nizamuddin station, where most of the Punjab trains had arrived. Before the 1950s, Lodi Road formed the southern tip of the capital; beyond it were 'open fields, where jackals howled and black bucks roamed'. On this reorganized land was our home, simply called 'J', the central nerve for a sprawling, close-knit family of cousins, aunts, friends and friends of friends, who all treated my dad's home as an open house for sleepovers and Sunday meals.

My father insisted he was improving.

As proof, he stood in the doorway of his bedroom and waved to me to go back to my own apartment. 'I am much better, see, I am walking.' I took a photograph of that moment that I haven't been able to look at again, since his death.

On the eighth day, his condition deteriorated and his fever spiked. The doctors said they would prefer him to be admitted to hospital. For us this was not an easy decision; for one we would be isolating him and leaving him alone. But we went by medical advice. How would we get a room, though? It was the end of April, and the wave was a tsunami.

From this moment on I became the news I had reported all these months. From begging for space in hospital to the anxiety over falling oxygen to researching the pros and cons of remdesivir, I was suddenly telling the COVID story in the first person.

Naresh Trehan, the celebrated surgeon, generously agreed that my dad could be brought to a general room at Medanta, the hospital he helmed. I convinced my reluctant father that we had to leave home by assuring him that he had permission to keep his own nursing attendant overnight, since he was not being admitted to the ICU. I promised him that once a series of tests was done, I would bring him home in two days.

I failed to keep my word.

On Tuesday morning, on 20 April, my father climbed down the steps of our home in crumpled blue pyjamas, taking the help of the polished wooden railing to slowly make his way down, shrugging off even then the help of the attendant. He was due for his second vaccine shot that very week.

The hospital's ambulances were busy till the afternoon. We panicked and, in what became one of the many decisions I have come to regret, started hunting for a private vehicle.

When the 'ambulance' arrived it turned out to be an old Maruti van that had been repurposed for the task. It had a crew of one; the driver and no accompanying paramedics. I glanced at the back. There was no stretcher, just the hard, flat grey slab of a worn-out seat. My eye travelled to an oxygen cylinder on the floor. Does it work, I asked the driver. He assured me it did. Then he suddenly asked me if we could provide the mask for oxygen. Suspicious of the infrastructure, I told him we would not travel with him if he was not fully equipped with a kit to administer the oxygen. He produced a mask and guaranteed me that everything was in order. By now, caught between panic and fear, I decided to take the chance and not lose more time. We helped our father on to the back. I sat in the front seat with the driver.

Along the way we encountered random police checkposts every few kilometres, set up to enforce the city's lockdown. They perilously slowed down a stream of ambulances, leading to a traffic snarl that could have made the difference between life and death. The driver had no idea of how to get to Medanta, and so I had one eye on Google Maps, another on my father at the back. 'Is he breathing,' I repeatedly asked his nurse. Over the noise of the traffic and the rickety vehicle we were in, my father motioned his hand at me in a wave, as if to say everything will be all right.

But by the time we reached the Medanta ICU my father's

oxygen levels after an hour of being on a cylinder had plummeted. The young doctor on the emergency shift told me that the mask fixed to the cylinder had not administered high-flow oxygen as it ought to have and my father was no longer in any condition to be admitted to a room as we had promised him. He needed to go straight to the ICU. And, naturally, there was no bed free immediately. My father was extricated from that sham of an ambulance, placed in a wheelchair, wheeled into the open lobby of the hospital and given a different oxygen cylinder. I stroked his hair and hugged him; he was barely conscious or cognizant of his surroundings. He had aged ten years in that hour. He sat hunched over, his hands limp, his face impassive.

Even in that horrific moment, when my heart was quite literally in my throat, I knew that my upper-class privilege, my relative access to monetary and other resources, made my father luckier than many Indians. After all, this is what I had spent months and months doing – telling the stories of those who were dying at the gates of hospitals, sometimes on the streets, because the healthcare system had crumbled.

Now I was on the other side; I was the protagonist instead of the chronicler. It was surreal, but also debilitating. I was so much more used to asking the questions, offering empathy, reflecting the rage. Suddenly, as the protagonist of my own sadness, I did not know how to cope.

That day was the last day I would see my father alive.

Over the next two days I managed only a crackly Facetime call with him on the doctor's mobile. Dad was hard of hearing and often used to piece together what we were saying by reading our lips. Unable to talk or hear and visibly uncomfortable with all the contraptions strapped to him, he formed a half sentence: 'I am choking, treat me.'

The hospital's doctors tried their best and I shall forever be grateful for that.

My father used to be an Air India executive in the glory years of the airline. Unlike his more contrarian and confrontational daughters, he was a universally liked man with perfect people skills. But at heart he was really a man of science. He walked out of a secure, salaried job when we were still in college, to dabble with entrepreneurship and the stuff he really loved – mathematics, meccano, and making things with his hands. A geeky inventor, he sometimes pulled apart electronic gadgets just so that he could experience the joy of reassembling them. In the now-locked cupboard of his room, saved between sheaths of tissue, is a newspaper clipping from his years in Modern School. It's a six-column story on the brilliant young boy who made a rocket that actually worked. As a young adult he built a vending machine for Cadbury chocolates well before the concept had arrived in India. We preserved it in our home with the love and awe one might feel for a museum piece. Over the years we stopped noticing it because it literally became part of the furniture. But I remember it vividly: white, curved at four edges, it looked like a small refrigerator, except for a black scrawl across its middle, one that tantalizingly promised a chocolate bar would drop out from its belly, in exchange for an inserted 25 paise coin.

Later he dabbled with other inventions, one of them a shoe-shine machine eponymously named 'Speedshine', used for some years by the posh Gymkhana Club. He was fascinated with the idea of creating a roti-maker. And there were his meccano pieces – trains, jet planes, ships that sailed on water, robots that talked. I would urge him to start a bespoke collection for commercial sales; he'd just laugh.

Speedy was so shaped by rationalism that when we were

growing up he urged my sister and me to either be entirely vegetarian from a love of animals or try every meat, including beef and pork.

In 2020, when the one-size-fits-all lockdown was announced – the one mistake the government learnt from and did not repeat or worsen in the sequel crisis – my father declared it to be an ill-thought move: 'Anyway, everyone is going to get it, sooner or later.'

I had reported from inside ICUs across the country. I had interviewed COVID-positive patients. I had been in crowded slums and buses and trucks. But as his daughter I could not meet my father; the hospital regulations forbade it. He had stopped reading my WhatsApp messages or writing any of his own. I scrawled a note for him and begged the nurse on duty to hand it over to him and to make sure he read it. I ended the note by telling him that we loved him and he would be back home with us shortly.

In the meanwhile, to keep myself focused – and somewhat sane – I kept working.

That same week, I went to report from a cremation ground in Old Delhi. A man sat on the street divider across the road from the grounds holding his head in his hands. Smoke clouds from the hundreds of burning pyres added grey to the blue evening sky. At the entrance, where 'Shamshan Ghat' was etched into the tiles, an unclaimed body wrapped in a white sheet lay on a metal stretcher. From the roof of the adjoining building all you could see were rows of bodies lined up to be burnt. The sky was overcast with orange and charcoal clouds. It was the colour of pain.

Inside, I met Jagdeep Singh, whose brother's body lay on the cold stone floor because the grounds had run out of space for the dead. Jagdeep Singh, in a wheelchair himself with one foot amputated because of diabetes, told me: 'When he was alive we couldn't offer him help; now that he is dead, we can't give him dignity. *Hum to bhagwan bharose reh gaye.* (We are now in God's hands.)' In the dimly lit grounds behind him, grieving relatives formed shadowy silhouettes against the blazing light of the pyres.

My agnostic heart said a silent prayer to God, thinking of my father, an atheist by temperament, who, lying alone in the ICU, did not even have God for solace.

There were many errors that the government would make in its response to the crisis – some from ignorance and incompetence and others from complacency and callousness. But what tied it all together for the citizens of our country was the sense of being orphaned. Many of us were bereaved after we lost parents to COVID. But if we had any expectation that the state would be benevolent, parental and empathetic, that hope was shattered. Whether in the first year, when millions of migrant workers were left to fend for themselves in a displacement so gigantic that it saw more people move than they had since Partition; or in the second wave, when Indians turned to each other for oxygen and beds, for drugs and blood donations, rarely bothering to tag official institutions of administration, aware all too keenly that this was a Darwinian struggle for survival and for support we only had each other.

One of my father's favourite phrases used to be: 'What cannot be cured, must be endured.' As a call to stoicism it was a great philosophy, even though, as my sister and I got older, we would sometimes snap at him, as adult children do, for talking to us the same way in our forties as he did when we were fourteen. When the lab confirmed he had COVID, I, desperate to buy time till I could think clearly, contemplated not telling him for a day. Ever tech savvy, he had already logged on and checked his own results by the time I could clear the fog in my head. He repeated his favourite phrase.

But it was misapplied.

My father, like hundreds of thousands of Indians, should not have had to endure what he did.

My father did not have to die.

Of course, I kept second-guessing my own decisions, right from my call to the ambulance to the very decision of not keep treating him at home. At least that way he'd have gone surrounded by the people who loved him. It's the thought of him all alone in his dying hours that is the most shattering.

But I also keep obsessing over whether a reduced gap between the two shots could have saved his life.

By May 2021, the UK, for instance, had reduced the gap between the required two vaccine shots from twelve to eight weeks. All new research showed that irrespective of which vaccine you took this time, a single shot did not offer as much protection against serious illness as two doses did; and the protection of a double shot was especially important when it came to symptomatic infections. A year on, with the advent of Omicron, the seventh variant of the virus, we now know that even two jabs are not enough to protect the elderly.

The May timeline would have been too late for my father. But I do keep thinking – had India just rolled out its vaccines sooner, had the government just ordered more vaccines earlier, had my father been double vaxxed, would he be alive today?

When my father got his first shot we discussed travelling together to New York in a few months. The city was where, while on a posting, my father enrolled in school at NYU in pursuit of his first love, maths. He'd cycle downtown on weekends for his master's in applied maths. His abiding regret was leaving his

PhD midway when he got transferred back to Delhi. We were excited about returning to our favourite city outside of home once he was safe and fully vaxxed.

Just like I can't bear to listen to music any more, I fear that travelling to the city he taught me how to ice-skate in may be just as traumatic.

When the dreaded call came at 3 a.m. from the night duty doctor at Medanta for my consent to place my father on the ventilator, I found myself unable to say no. I felt claustrophobic from fear; I ran out of my house and stood alone in the darkness of a desolate neighbourhood, under the white glow of a street light. I didn't have too much time to decide. All my theories about 'letting him go peacefully' came to naught in that instance. If there was even a 0.1 per cent chance of him making it, I was going to take it.

When we took his body from the hospital to the nearest cremation ground, I could not help but notice the irony. Now that he was dead, we had managed to organize a professional ambulance. The stretcher in the hearse was shiny brown, the leather was new, the height of the seat was adjustable. And there lay my father, who had at least a decade more left of life before COVID, in a beige zip bag, as if he were a frozen vegetable, lost to us forever. Speedy Dutt, he of the kind heart, maverick and liberal mind and twinkling eyes, died, a ventilator strapped to him in his final hours. Like every child anywhere during this pandemic I felt it was all my fault.

I stared at him for a long time through the glass of the ambulance and said a silent prayer to God, asking forgiveness for all the mistakes I had made – for the time I should have spent at home and didn't, for the moments that I snapped at him and shouldn't have, for the website I wanted to start in his name and never did and for the ambulance I should never have taken him to hospital in.

Our trauma did not end there. At the funeral ground three other families had been given the same 'token' and time slot as us. An argument ensued; there were raised voices, threats, shouting and screaming, a near-fisticuffs situation. Usually, I'm a scrapper. This time I sat quietly on a bench, looking at the bodies precariously placed on mountains of wood, one after the other, for as long as the eye could see, and let my sister handle the confrontation.

Eventually we sought the help of the police to cremate my father.

By the time I got back home I had a fever. By evening I was COVID positive.

The sickness compounded the grief and yet stood in its way.

As my smell and taste slipped away from me and my fever spiked, I did not know if COVID was numbing me against my loss or just displaying its usual symptoms. I lost the ability to separate the physical manifestations of my COVID from my broken-down mental state. Overanxious doctors advised a double dose of steroids to break my fever. Soon after, the overuse of dexamethasone, by now the standard steroid in India's clinical management of the virus, was ferociously contested. That it was deployed so readily even in mild and moderate cases was linked to the sudden outbreak of 'black fungus', or mucormycosis, a rare fungal infection, often characterized by a swollen, bulging eye that could lead to loss of vision. In horror, I watched my face, arms and feet balloon from the steroids. And my hair started to fall off in clumps, an experience so many people had in the aftermath of COVID. But all of it felt like a blur; it felt as if the centre of gravity had shifted and left me straggling behind, unable to find my balance.

And since then, I, who think of myself as iron-framed, tough and fazed by little, have been too terrified to step into my father's bedroom, where his meccano trains run on three white rail tracks that he affixed to the roof of his room so that if you glanced up at any point you would see all of his magnificent and colourful creations. Under his bed, sacks of meccano parts lay scattered across the floor untidily. In one corner, his Mac desktop, on which he would spend hours surfing, gathered dust. On the wall behind where he sat once, his wife's portrait in black and white captures a woman throwing her head back and laughing uproariously.

I don't really know if the room is like this even now.

This is how it is in my memory – the three music systems, including an ancient, decrepit eight-track, the ironing board that had been converted into a repairs workshop table for clocks and toasters and ovens that no longer worked and needed fixing, the storeroom with dozens of suitcases, all packed with more meccano parts that he would order from all across the world, the cupboards packed with suits and shirts that he barely ever wore, and of course the rail tracks that came sliding down from the roof making his bedroom feel like a mad hatter's den. Just before he got COVID he had proudly showed me a cuckoo clock that he had managed to revive.

I do not know when I shall have the courage to step into my father's room. I am frightened of what it may make me feel.

Eight months after his death I was still scared.

I wasn't scared of the virus as I travelled more than 30,000 kilometres by road across India through the first wave, and then again thousands of kilometres by both air and road through the more lethal second spell. During both the first national lockdown and the localized shutdowns of the second year, I became the chronicler of death and despair – from hospitals, cremation grounds and graveyards; from slums and tenements where social distancing was an impossibility, from crowded trucks and trains and also from the inside of ICUs crumbling under the weight of COVID, till eventually, and ironically, there was no separation left between me and the subject I was covering. We had become one.

It was never the COVID that triggered my fear.

It was – and remains – the fear of confronting loss.

The only thing that helps sometimes is giving voice to the perspective and suffering of others.

What could be worse than a daughter losing her parents?

Possibly, parents losing their children.

In Meerut, at St Luke's Church, as the nuns of the church said their prayers in the garden, I strolled to the back where the cemetery is to find two graves dressed in marigold ribbons. They were the graves of Joefred and Ralphred, identical twins, sons of schoolteachers Gregory Raymond and Soja Raphael. Both engineers had turned twenty-four a day before they tested positive, just a few weeks ago on 23 April. Bound together in life, they were now together in death. Gregory, the son of a soldier, told me that the moment Joefred died, he would lose his other son too. Though they kept the news from Ralphred, the twins always had a sixth sense about each other. They died within hours of each other.

There were two roses, one for each brother, at their graves.

At home in Delhi, sixteen days after my infection and isolation, I took my father's ashes, mixed them into the mud of a rose plant, sat on the cement floor, folded my hands in gratitude and helplessness, and set off for the road again. Soon, I was back on the reporting trail in the remotest interiors of rural India. Not because COVID had not been debilitating – actually it was like no other sickness I have ever experienced – but because after my father died I knew of no other way to cope with the cavernous emptiness inside me than to redouble my commitment to the telling of this tragedy.

My grief feels personal, yet universal.

After my father's death my life felt even more consumed by COVID than before.

I have become obsessed with the telling of this tale.

In COVID's story is also his story.

The impact of the Delta variant in the months of April and May 2021 was so devastating it literally left India gasping for breath. Within a fortnight the demand for medical oxygen tripled. Because of the fast-acting virulence of Delta and the short time span within which it erupted, 54.5 per cent of those hospitalized needed assisted oxygen in the second wave, in contrast to 41.1 per cent in the first wave within a fortnight of its eruption.[25] Transporting oxygen by air was complicated as it was inflammable. Slow-moving oxygen tankers needed to move from the east of the country right across to the north and west. In the absence of any other effective therapeutic treatment, high-flow oxygen was the only way to prolong lives in the ICU. But dozens of hospitals across states ran short of oxygen, leading to mass deaths. These deaths were never acknowledged as being related to the shortage of oxygen. But eyewitness testimonies are detailed, comprehensive and unequivocal.

9

Asphyxiated

On the night of 23 April 2021, at around 8.30 p.m., Sherchand, a daily wage employee at the Municipal Corporation of Delhi, squeezed into pale green scrubs borrowed from a nurse he had befriended, tied a scarf over his head, wore a simple three-tier surgical mask across his face and entered the ICU of the Jaipur Golden Hospital, where his wife had been battling COVID for the last seven days.

Unlike several hospitals that were extremely stringent about treating the virus as an isolation illness and barred relatives from meeting patients, Jaipur Golden was somewhat more flexible. Its promoters were the family of Sardari Lal Bahri, a refugee family from Pakistan whose wealth had been built on the back of a hugely successful transport and trucking company. That day the 250-bed hospital, a 'multi-speciality' facility, was packed to capacity.

'*Yeh meri Manju begum hai, meri madam ko corona ho gaya hai,*' (This is my darling Manju. She has corona now) Sherchand said, smiling into the camera, flicking it to selfie mode. 'But I am helping her and she will be better soon.' One hand was outstretched to hold the phone, the other formed a protective hook around his wife, who was breathing into a mask she held with both hands, as if life itself depended on it. 'If we have to beat corona, we have to first banish our fear,' Sherchand went on cheerfully, convinced that the tide had turned, the worst was over and he'd be able to take his wife home soon. He blew kisses at her and watched her cheeks turn pink from behind the pipes and tubes.

'She was embarrassed about the flying kisses,' said Sherchand, sitting cross-legged on the floor of his bare, furniture-less flat, amid a small pile of drawing books, smiling at the memory of his wife's coyness as he flipped through their wedding album. Manju, posing in glittery bridal red, standing somewhat self-consciously against a shiny studio wall, smiled right back.

Sherchand would often spend long hours in the hospital canteen. He would sleep several nights in the small public garden in front of the building so that he could be close at hand to 'my madam'. Their three children were left in the care of relatives.

He was feeling especially hopeful that day. The doctors had told him Manju was getting better; they had asked him to procure an injection of tocilizumab, an immunosuppressive drug normally used in the treatment of rheumatoid arthritis, a single vial of which cost anywhere between ₹40,000 and ₹50,000. Private hospitals across India were asking desperate relatives to make their own arrangements to procure it and black marketeers had already pushed the price to as high as ₹200,000 in some cities. Sherchand's only worry that evening was how to manage the money. On his monthly salary of ₹13,000, he would not have been able to pay even one day of the hospital fees. To get Manju treated he had already run through most of his life savings. The bills were being paid from the distress sale of a small plot of land in his village that he had originally hoped would allow him to purchase a small house and live rent-free in the city. 'I would have done anything to save my wife,' he told me.

An hour or so after he met his wife that evening, he was sipping on a cup of tea when he saw people running helter-skelter near the hospital reception. In the distance, he could hear people shouting in panic. He overheard snatches of incomplete conversation from hospital staff, who mentioned oxygen shortage. He saw some people rushing in and racing ahead with a single oxygen cylinder held in their arms, desperately making their way past the swelling crowd.

Sherchand was not on social media. So he didn't know that the hospital had taken to Twitter with a dire warning about its oxygen supply running short.

Pushing his way through the melee of people, some crying, some angry, Sherchand managed to make his way inside the ICU again. Manju was gasping for breath, but still alive. Sherchand counted at least four bodies in the ward before the guard shouted at him and pushed him out. Outside, through tears, he dialled his nephew and his wife's family telling them to get to the hospital as fast as they could.

By then there were police swarming the premises. Families initially thought the police had arrived to make an intervention on their behalf. Perhaps a patient's family had complained. But they soon discovered that the police had been summoned to 'control' them. As the day entered the wee hours of the morning and as more and more people got the much-dreaded phone call from the hospital, the police were in fact there, at the request of the hospital, to contain possible violence on the part of distraught relatives.

Among those waiting at the hospital reception that night were sisters Navya and Prachi Awasthi. Their mother's last message to them earlier in the day had been about mangoes. Seema Awasthi, school principal, fifty-six years old, wanted her favourite safeda to be cut into smaller pieces instead of the clunky portions packed into her tiffin every day. The message made her daughters laugh. Mum was getting better; even the doctors said so. That morning, on his rounds, the doctor on ICU duty even showed the family proof. Seema's oxygen levels, derailed by the Delta variant of the virus, were on the rise again, in the high 80s when unassisted and in the late 90s when she was placed on the non-invasive-ventilation mask (NIV).

The girls showed me their favourite picture of Seema – a wide, toothy smile splitting her face and mehndi-patterned flowers dressing her arms from palm to elbow. She seemed to be dancing with an abandon that only someone who has embraced life in full can. Seema was determined to get better and get back to the job she loved and the daughters she had raised as a single parent.

It was shortly after 10 p.m. when their aunt first got a phone call from the hospital. It was a security guard who was letting them know that Seema was being placed on a ventilator. They argued with the guard; a ventilator needed family consent; the hospital was not empowered to take this decision. But, unknown to the family, the oxygen crisis had unravelled chaos inside the ICU. The Awasthi sisters say they could not get a doctor on the phone.

The sisters scrambled to get to the hospital, where the receptionists on duty were turning away new COVID-positive patients who were begging for beds. They heard a 'weird beeping sound' somewhere in the background. 'It was a very weird vibe.'

Prachi and Navya were told their mother had suffered a

cardiac arrest. No one in the administration spoke about the oxygen shortage to them. But as they stood in the foyer of the hospital, overwhelmed and defeated, they witnessed an oxygen tanker driving into the premises almost close to midnight. 'As a hospital it is your moral duty that when you realize that you don't have enough oxygen, you inform families instead of letting people die. Maybe we could have done something, maybe we could have found oxygen. They took away our right to life.'

Instead, the sisters discovered – and only after they joined a support group with other families – that in its discharge papers, the hospital not just omitted to mention the rupture in oxygen supply, it had also staggered the time of the deaths over several hours, to avoid their being linked to a single incident.

Managers of hospitals across India responded with similar opacity.

Earlier that day, twenty-five patients died within twenty-four hours at the prestigious Ganga Ram Hospital in the capital, considered one of the best medical facilities in India. Five hundred patients were being treated for COVID here, among whom 142 were on high-flow oxygen support. Ganga Ram has always enjoyed a prestigious legacy. Founded in 1921 in pre-Partition Lahore by the eponymous bureaucrat-engineer, its post-Independence branch was inaugurated in India by Jawaharlal Nehru in 1954. But the mighty fell too. Senior officials at the hospital contradicted each other over whether the mass deaths here had been a consequence of oxygen shortage. The medical director confirmed 'low oxygen concentration' as a likely cause of the deaths; the chairman said they had just happened to be 'our twenty-five sickest patients'. Both agreed that the ventilators and BiPAP machines in the ICUs, meant to stabilize the respiratory system and create a steady pattern of breathing among patients, were not working effectively. The lives of sixty more patients could be at risk if oxygen was not rushed to the hospital.

We were not allowed inside the Ganga Ram Hospital compound the morning after the catastrophe. But in the small public park across the road from the building, I met distraught relatives of patients who were still undergoing treatment inside, carrying small tanks of oxygen alongside flasks of tea and parathas wrapped in aluminium foils. Others carried oxygen concentrators, machines more suitable for home care. But those were all that was available in the market.

Six days later, on 29 April, another hospital sent an SOS out into the ether. Doctor Ubaid Hamid, the medical director at New Delhi's Vimhans Hospital, was in absolute panic because 170 of the 210 patients admitted were oxygen dependent. After several desperate pleas, a government tanker with 800 litres of oxygen had been dispatched, but the supply would last only another two hours.

For many families that wait would prove to be lethal.

Outside the hospital, sitting in the front seat of her parked Maruti car, her feet facing the pavement, Himanshi held her stomach and rocked her body back and forth. Her hair was dishevelled, her eyes blank from acute shock, her words incoherent. Her brother would lean forward and hold her and stroke her head gently to console her. But there was really nothing to be said.

'*Papa chale gaye.*' She kept repeating the sentence over and over again because its truth was so implausible and unpalatable. 'My father has gone.'

Her face had no make-up, and her short black-and-white kurta was crumpled, as if she had spent the night curled up in

Asphyxiated

the car. She pulled out a phone from her bag and showed it to us. 'Look, look here,' she said, almost shouting, 'this is his last WhatsApp message.'

Himanshi's father collapsed after a steep drop in the level of oxygen that was being given to him. When we started to tell Himanshi what explanation the hospital had offered, she interrupted angrily. '*Mar gaye hain.* He is dead.'

Her brother Puru opened the rear door with an abrupt angry wave of his hand. 'Look, we have not one, but two,' he said, as two cylinders of oxygen rolled on the back seat. 'We gave the hospital these cylinders. Even then they couldn't save him.'

Twenty-nine-year-old Himanshi, a software engineer, thought that by admitting her father to a private hospital she was keeping him safe. That afternoon, when she heard from her father for the very last time, Himanshi was at the government-run LNJP Hospital, where she had just managed to get her mother a bed with enormous difficulty. She raced to Ganga Ram as soon as she got his text.

The name of the family WhatsApp group – consisting of the three children and their parents – was 'Get Well Soon, Lucky!' For a while it seemed that that was exactly what would happen. The kids had been talking to their dad about whether they should send him some coconut water to drink. Anil Khanna, fifty-seven, a distributor in the FMCG business, wrote to his children at 3 p.m. saying, '*Yahan oxygen ki shortage hai. Lagta hai khatam ho gaya hai.*' (There is a shortage of oxygen here. Seems like nothing is left now.)

When Himanshi saw this message from her father, she wrote one word in response. 'Coming.'

Persistent messages from the siblings to their father after that went unread and unresponded to.

He died the same day.

India produces over 7,000 tonnes of oxygen every day, including for use by industries. Before the pandemic hit, only 15 per cent of this supply was used for medical purposes. Even till the second week of April, during the second wave, the daily need for medical oxygen was under 4,000 tonnes. It tripled within a fortnight as COVID cases surged, from 3,842 metric tonnes per day on 12 April to 8,400 metric tonnes daily by 25 April. By the first week of May, the requirement had soared to 11,000 metric tonnes every day.[26] The failure to anticipate the second wave – and thus the demand for high-flow oxygen – resulted in a man-made crisis.

Oxygen is not produced uniformly across the country; eight states, most of them in the north and east, account for 80 per cent of the country's oxygen production. Ferrying of inflammable material comes with its own challenges. With a temperature of minus 183 degrees Celsius, liquid oxygen, a cryogenic gas, cannot be airlifted. It takes up to two hours to fill one tanker, and oxygen tankers are instructed to move at no faster a speed than 40 kilometres per hour. Tankers were now required to travel several hundred kilometres. So, even when the government insisted that the production capacity in the country was sufficient to meet the pandemic's soaring demands, the large expanse across which the oxygen had to be transported and the difficulty in moving cryogenic material resulted in fatal delays. In many instances, oxygen had to be moved right across the breadth of India – from the east, where it was produced in surplus for giant steel factories, to the west, which was most severely hit by the virus. By the third week of April more than half of those admitted to hospital – that is, one in every two patients – needed to be treated with oxygen support. That was a nearly 14 per cent increase over the requirement in the first wave.

'What's happening is murder, not natural death from a pandemic,' said Arokaiaswamy Velumani, scientist and promoter of Thyrocare laboratories, as hospital after hospital shut their doors to patients because their ICUs turned non-functional in the absence of guaranteed oxygen supply.

Eight months after the onset of COVID in India, in October 2020, the health ministry invited competitive bids to build oxygen plants in hospital premises. The plan was focused on pressure swing adsorption (PSA) plants, which can absorb nitrogen from the air at nearly ambient temperatures. While oxygen 'trapped' in this form is not considered as effective as liquid oxygen from cryogenic technology, there's no question that it would have helped in containing the humanitarian crisis. But as of April 2021, as people began to die on the streets outside hospital gates that had been closed to them, and sometimes in ambulances that ran short of oxygen, only thirty-three such plants out of the 162 that were sanctioned had been built. Money from the PM Cares Fund was allotted only in January, and by the time the worst of the second wave was upon India the crisis was too large to contain.

Maharashtra, the state that is the largest producer of oxygen in India in peacetime, was the first to run short as it had the largest number of COVID cases. It was early April when doctors in Mumbai began to sound the alarm and warn the rest of the country about what was coming. 'We can do without remdesivir and tocilizumab, but we cannot manage without oxygen, we are on tenterhooks,' said Dr Swaroop Hegde at the city's SRV Hospital, where in the second week of April it was already down to 10 per cent of regular supply. Hegde explained that treatment inside ICU wards would have to change – high-flow cannulas would be the first to go, and if normal COVID treatment demanded oxygen supply at 10 litres per minute per patient, that would now have to come down to something like 3 litres per minute. Patients who were critical (and thus in need of more high-flow oxygen) would have to be turned away. 'The entire line of treatment is compromised. This can mean only one thing – more deaths.'

At smaller hospitals, where mostly poorer citizens were treated, the situation was even more dire. In Chembur, the Mumbai suburb built on reclamation land and said to be named after *chemburee*, the Marathi word for crab, the twenty-five-bed Sai Hospital was already treating thirty-three patients, with patients sometimes doubling up on beds. Every afternoon, ward boys and attendants who should have been looking after the ailing would hop on to a small lorry and drive for up to an hour across the highway to the harbour town of Turbhe to purchase as many oxygen cylinders as they could find from vendors, who in turn often had to source them from black marketeers. Then at the hospital they would unload the cylinders, one at a time, rolling them on the uneven stone ground till they could nudge them inside the cramped little elevator up to the sickest patients.

Among the earliest deaths from oxygen deficiency at a hospital in India happened on the outskirts of Mumbai in the Vasai–Palghar belt, just an hour's drive from the international airport. On 13 April, policemen swarmed outside the private Vinayak Hospital in the emerging industrial town of Nalasopara. A woman sat on the faux plastic chair in the waiting area outside, holding her head in her hands. Next to her, a relative reached out to hold her close. They sat in absolute silence. Inside, below a statue of Ganesha garlanded with marigolds and a portrait of Lord Krishna just above the elephant god, stony-faced hospital staff declined to answer any questions and shooed us out of the premises. The evening before, enraged families had come to blows with the administrative staff as the news of eleven deaths, all within a few hours of each other, trickled out.

Ram Babu Tailor, as everyone called him, was in that list of eleven. At home, in a small room in the matchbox-sized apartments that are stacked up in narrow columns, his wife, son and daughter sat on the floor of a bare room, in wordless grief. On a high table in the same room, occupying pride of place, was Ram Babu's sewing machine. One wall was plastered with portraits of gods – Durga, Krishna, Shiva; on another, a clock hung lopsidedly, as if time itself had gone all topsy-turvy. Ram Babu was only fifty-two. His wife Rekha said they had already run up a bill of ₹150,000 and had dipped into the life savings that they had kept aside for the weddings of their children. Ram Babu's son Rahul got a call from the hospital informing him that his father was 'critical'. Inside the ward Rahul saw the other patients already draped from head to toe in sheets that were now shrouds. His father was being intubated; doctors said there was a 1 per cent chance he may make it. Minutes later he was dead.

The deaths in Nalasopara in early April should have sounded the alarm for the rest of the country. It provided enough time for the supply chain and logistics for oxygen distribution to be worked out. The military could have been deployed to handle this nationwide operational emergency. After all, the army had extensive experience in moving men and machines at short notice, building temporary bridges over flood waters and running convoys from centralized war rooms. Instead, as states desperate to keep the oxygen for themselves bickered and fought, tankers were held up for hours at provincial borders by local police.

And three weeks after the deaths at Vinayak Hospital, the same nightmare unfolded in hospital after hospital across India.

'Oximeter, oximeter, someone give her an oximeter.' Rishab, a young man in his twenties, brought his car to a screeching halt as he pulled up outside a gurudwara in Indirapuram in Uttar Pradesh. He was in tears, trembling and gasping in panic as his seventy-seven-year-old grandmother lay hunched over in a listless heap in the back seat, her shoulders drooping and head leaning to one side. On the street outside the gurudwara, which normally fed kada prasad to the hungry, people had lined up all along the length of the pavement for an oxygen 'langar'. From giant cylinders all along the stretch of the main road, tubes and pipes were hooked up to men and women, most of them elderly, sitting inside vehicles, allowing them up to thirty minutes of respite from breathlessness. It was a drive-through oxygen arcade set up to help those who could not get admission to hospital. Volunteers rushed a cylinder to Rishab's car. His grandmother leaned back in the seat, finally able to breathe, as another relative stroked her head gently. From the distance, all you could see was her grey hair gleaming in the dark under the dim glow of a street lamp. In the shadowy evening light, some lay flat on wrought-iron benches outside the gurudwara, others sat stoically in plastic chairs placed in a single-file row. Even private ambulances, mostly stocked with a single cylinder that could last no longer than a few hours, came here for help.

Every morning, Sikhs who had signed up to assist the gurudwara in running the langar would carry away their now-empty cylinders to be refilled.

But this inspirational spirit of *sewa* could only offer

temporary relief; a hospital still had to be found. Most of those who turned to the oxygen langar came after trying their luck at a half dozen hospitals. Rishab and his grandmother had driven to Indirapuram after visiting half a dozen hospitals, including Guru Teg Bahadur (GTB) Hospital, one of Delhi's main government facilities.

At GTB, like so many hospitals that month, security guards stood like bouncers at the firmly shut gates. All questions were redirected to an A-4-sized printout pasted untidily on the wall. With limited oxygen supply, GTB was taking no chances. It had closed its doors to new patients.

Outside, a young man stood near an autorickshaw on the road holding a one-day-old baby wrapped in a fluffy, patterned blanket. At the back of the rickshaw, a woman in a pink nightie sat with her legs slightly parted to manage the weight her slender frame had been carrying all these months. While the mother, Rachna, was being operated upon at a hospital ten kilometres away for the delivery of her baby, the mandatory tests had shown that she was also COVID positive. Vaccines for pregnant women had not yet been approved, so she'd had no protection through her nine months. The hospital referred them to GTB, and an ambulance dropped them off on the road and sped away. Rachna's husband made an SOS call to his father, an autorickshaw driver, who met them at the hospital gates. Her day-old newborn infant was placed in the care of relatives. The lack of oxygen had forced the hospital's hand. There was no bed available for Rachna. Oxygen-supported beds increased fourfold from the first wave to the second, according to government data, going from 62,000 in April 2020 up to 270,000 in March 2021. This number stood at 425,000 in July 2021. The number of ventilators available increased from

14,400 to 57,518 between March 2020 and July 2021. But despite this huge increase, as Delta ripped through the health system, it all fell calamitously short.[27]

As Rachna lay sprawled out and helpless on the shiny green rexine seat of her father-in-law's autorickshaw, next to the vehicle, in the back seat of a white sedan, Lovely struggled to breathe. She was panting and heaving and in acute distress. She had tested positive for COVID but could not get medical care anywhere. She pulled her face mask down and lay back against the leather while her son tried to negotiate with the security guards at the barricaded entrance. As he pleaded with them his phone rang incessantly. There was a funeral to be organized and the extended family had a million questions and queries. Lovely did not know it then, but her husband had died earlier that day at another public hospital in the city. Desperate relatives hit the SOS button when Deepak Kumar Sharma, who had been trying to recuperate in home isolation, told them he was finding it difficult to breathe. They went to at least four hospitals; finally, after speaking with someone the family knew in the chief minister's office, they were able to persuade staff at the RML Hospital to let their car in. By the time the guards opened the gates Deepak had already died.

No official separate count has been done of the thousands of Indians, maybe more, who died – not from the virus – but from the deficit of oxygen. These 'oxygen deaths' must include not only those who perished in ICUs where assisted breathing machines suddenly went cold, but must also count and acknowledge those who died out on the streets, in the back of cars and on motorcycles or waiting long hours in ambulances, all because an inadequate oxygen supply reduced the bed capacity of hospitals, forcing them to turn patients away.

Asphyxiated

During the second wave, the production and movement of oxygen became a mammoth warlike operation precisely because it was treated as a sudden invasion instead of as an anticipated threat. In fact, what was needed was not an over-centralized, pan-India intervention; had there been a series of small, localized, commonsensical measures taken a few months prior, there would have likely been no deaths from an oxygen shortfall.

A tribal district in Maharashtra showed how it could be done. While India's cities were asphyxiated, Nandurbar, identified as one of the 250 most backward districts of India, with a literacy rate of under 64 per cent, became a model for oxygen management. Its collector, Rajendra Bharud, a medical doctor before he became a civil servant, demonstrated that India's oxygen deaths were entirely preventable, and that is exactly what made them almost akin to murder.

Nandurbar is situated along Maharashtra's borders with Madhya Pradesh and Gujarat with the mighty Narmada river framing its northern edges. Poverty and remoteness have left Nandurbar without the benefits of medical infrastructure that other parts of the country have. Bharud's job was to find a way to minimize deaths in an area that did not have a single multi-speciality hospital or medical college. He calculated that only 10 per cent of COVID patients would be serious enough to need oxygen; everyone else could be treated in isolation centres. To make sure that oxygenated beds would not run short, Bharud commissioned an oxygen plant in the district at a cost of ₹8,50,000. By the time the second wave lashed against the shores of Nandurbar, the facility was manufacturing 125 jumbo cylinders of oxygen daily. Every minute, 2,000 litres of oxygen was being produced at this plant. As COVID cases began to spiral in America and Brazil, Bharud convinced private companies to add plants in the district. Nandurbar had three oxygen plants and a surplus of oxygenated beds towards the end of April when the rest of the country was still waiting to exhale.

Bharud had grown up in poverty and was raised by a single mother, his father having died when Kamalabai was pregnant with him. One of three children whose family had to sell local wine made from mahua flowers to make ends meet, Bharud could never shake off the memory of the thatched roof they had lived under in his childhood, one that was assembled from sugarcane straw. Bharud, who does not know what his father looked like – his parents were too poor to ever get anyone to click a photograph, and this was the age before smartphones became ubiquitous – believes his early hardships made him more sensitive to the despair of marginalized communities. Little did he know that he would come to be a global illustration of how effective governance could make all the difference between life and death in a pandemic. Nandurbar still had to battle a high mortality rate because of a shortage of doctors at the primary healthcare centres, delayed hospital admissions and acute vaccine hesitancy among its rural residents. But it was among the best-managed districts in the country in terms of oxygen management, underscoring how preventable the crisis was.

In other parts of the country, the situation spiralled out of control so terribly that in a modern-day version of signing your own death warrant, families were asked to sign waivers that would exempt the hospital from all responsibility if a death were to take place there on account of shortage of oxygen.

At Delhi's Ambedkar Hospital, twenty-one-year-old Jatin Kumar waited by the ambulance for his father Manoj Kumar's body to be released by the hospital authorities. Starved of oxygen, the hospital had to ration its use. Jatin had to literally beg them to administer oxygen to his father in the ICU. Now that his father, a fifty-three-year-old businessman, was dead, there was nothing he could do but rage. He had put his signature on a consent form that signed away not just all decision-making to the doctors on duty, but also forfeited his right to take legal action against the hospital for the meagre supply of oxygen and any fatality as a consequence of that. The women of the family stood around the body, sobbing into their flimsy blue masks. The men, more stoic, had a piece of advice for others: 'Do not come to hospital if you have COVID, coming to hospital is like coming to die. You will die if you come to a hospital.'

That was cynicism and pain speaking. And doctors argued that they were victims who had been vilified. Five minutes of interruption in the oxygen pipeline can mean brain damage or death for a patient strapped to it, explained Dr Sudhanshu Bankata, who watched both patients and colleagues suffer at Batra Hospital in the capital. A doctor was among the twelve lives lost on the night of 1 May in the ICU. 'We want to compete with Beijing and Tokyo but don't have enough oxygen. We needed 6.5 metric tonnes every day and were being provided 4.2 metric tonnes. When things became critical we reached out to every channel, every digital platform, begged, cried and did everything we could, but by the time the oxygen tankers came, it was too late,' he said, recalling the night of 'sheer misery and utter desperation'.

Health workers at the front line were certainly not responsible for the shortage – more than one broke down in videos that went viral, and others called it the worst day of their medical careers. But there were grave questions about how cash-rich managements of hospitals had handled the oxygen catastrophe.

Guidelines stipulated by the Indian Council of Medical

Research asked for hospital documents to classify deaths as COVID or non-COVID and allowed for no further stratification. As a result, several hospitals across India where lack of oxygen was the cause of patient deaths issued discharge slips that described the deaths as a 'consequence of respiratory failure'.

'We were robbed. We were robbed of our mother's life, we were robbed of the chance to save her and now we have been robbed of justice,' said Prachi Awasthi, as the families mobilized to go to court. 'And the doctors who remained silent and watched the hospitals do this broke their oath.'

But the doctors were just as despairing. 'What did all the thalis and taalis amount to,' said Bankata, referencing the prime minister's call for symbolic national solidarity during the first wave. 'We were losing patients one by one. We felt like the emperor who had no clothes. Our promises were empty.'

On 20 July, the government informed Parliament that no death had taken place in the country as a result of oxygen shortage. The Centre had collated this information based on the information sent by states, and no state reported any such death.

On the same day, I met Shalu Kataria in her home in Naraina village in south-west Delhi. Despite being in the lap of the capital's Central Ridge line – an expanse of reserved forest land – this area had been ignored on all key development indices. You could only drive up to the gate, from where you had to get off and walk through cobbled lanes and a haphazardly organized web of small plots with narrow constructions.

A corridor opened up to a room where Shalu's father-in-law lay asleep and unwell on a single bed. Shalu guided us up sharp steep steps to a terrace where we sat, her two children and I, against white sacks of Ambuja cement, and spoke of that fateful day that her husband died. Her children, Yasmin and Ruben, were only eleven and six years old.

Dinesh Kataria, forty-one, was among the patients admitted to Jaipur Golden Hospital. The day before his death the hospital had asked Shalu to organize for plasma therapy for her husband. Though plasma therapy was dropped by August 2021 as an approved intervention for the clinical management of COVID, at the very peak of the second wave, families of patients would desperately be hunting for plasma donors. The technique essentially involved using a component of blood from a recovered COVID patient as therapy on one who was still ill. It was one of the many half-baked, unproven measures applied with great fanfare through those hellish few months, and though on paper it was meant to be donation-driven, poor patients sometimes ended up paying hundreds of thousands of rupees to organize for plasma.

Shalu, a deceptively frail-looking woman with a pencil-thin frame and jet-black hair, hugged her children close as she spoke to me. After the plasma was organized, the hospital wanted to administer tocilizumab to her husband. By now the injection was referred to as the rich man's drug – *'ameer logon ki dawai'*. I had lost count of the number of people who had taken loans just to purchase this high-end treatment or, worse, remdesivir that was being sold illegally at prices twenty times higher than its official cost. Remdesivir was later dropped from all advisory guidelines. This is what made the oxygen-shortage deaths especially egregious; patients and their families had already been left to fend for themselves.

Shalu was in a quandary. The injection was more expensive by nearly ₹15,000 if bought from the hospital; she was trying to find a supplier outside. The family was already paying off the debt on a loan of ₹2,000,000. The doctors said Dinesh was steady, and underlined that with medical assistance his oxygen levels were showing a decent saturation of 95. Shalu was allowed to meet him for a few minutes and she took a photograph of him picking at his lunch of dal, rice and yogurt.

At this point, Shalu's voice broke. She had to pause to comfort her daughter, whose eyes were welling up with tears. When she gathered strength and resumed recounting the tragedy, Shalu told me she did not go home that night; she was anxious and waited downstairs in a common waiting area. A little after 11 p.m. that night, Dinesh rang Shalu and asked her to rush upstairs.

But the guard wouldn't let her in. Nothing worked, neither tears nor cajoling.

Shalu lied that she needed to use the toilet, which she knew was past the security barricade. As soon as she crossed it, she rushed towards her husband's bed in the ICU. She saw a cloth partition had been placed to provide a covering and doctors were leaning over his bed manually pumping his chest. She ran towards his bed; his hands and feet were icy cold. The doctors asked her to step back.

Half an hour later, at midnight, the hospital officially told her Dinesh had died.

There was chaos in the corridors and angry and grieving relatives. But even at this hour Shalu was not aware that the oxygen supply to the hospital had been interrupted. It was only the next morning when she saw relatives arrive at the compound carrying cylinders in their arms that she processed the magnitude of what had occurred.

Shalu was sobbing as she spoke. This time it was her daughter who held her mother close and motioned to her to keep going.

'*Kya se kya ho gaya, hamari duniya khatam ho gayee hai,*' (Our world has ended) sobbed Shalu into her mask. 'If they could ask me to organize injections and plasma, could they not have asked me to organize oxygen? I would have got them oxygen, I would have made sure my husband lived. I feel manipulated. I was all alone, I didn't understand what was happening. If only the guard had let me see him earlier, maybe I would have at least seen him alive.'

Anxiety for the future deepened her grief. Shalu did not have money to pay her children's school fees that month; a request for a waiver had been denied. She was terrified that her children would be thrown out of school.

A few days later, Yasmin and Ruben Kataria petitioned the Delhi High Court demanding answers – and justice. They were children who spoke for an entire nation.

The images of the summer of 2021 were unprecedented. Bodies had stacked up all along the banks of the river Ganga in Uttar Pradesh and Bihar. In Madhya Pradesh, undertakers at cremation sites ran out of wood. In the prime minister's constituency of Varanasi, bodies were washed ashore. In Rajasthan, an officer who issued death certificates could not get one for his own wife who had died from COVID. Amidst a raging controversy over exactly how many Indians died during the pandemic, a combination of factors converged to uncount the dead. The actual number of deaths likely runs into millions, and if so, makes the pandemic the biggest human tragedy in India since Partition.

10

'Awaaz De Kahan Hai'

Mashkoor Mohammed Khan sat hunched over a small metal box of trinkets, his back forming a listless concave curve on the charpoy. His cloth mask had slid down to his chin. And as he held his white-haired head in his hands, he wept.

From a little compartment in the box he pulled out a photograph of the woman who used to sleep by his side, on a separate bed in recent years, in the open courtyard of their small village in central Madhya Pradesh. 'She used to lie just here, and look over me all night,' he motioned towards the adjacent space. Where there was once a person, there was a green trunk now, balanced on two bricks. It was pushed against a locked aluminium door with a faded brown duster slung over it. Then he pointed to a picture so tiny he had to hold it between his thumb and index finger. 'That's Fatima.'

His wife wore a deep-maroon hijab over her head as she looked straight into the camera with a steely, determined gaze.

'I am broken,' he said, barely able to form words through tears, his entire frame convulsed with grief. *'Main toot gaya, mera sab kuch khatam ho gaya. Sab kuch.*' (Everything that mattered to me is gone.)

Mashkoor had not risen from his bed in days. Wearing a crumpled white kurta over a blue printed lungi, he folded one leg under him and showed us more pictures. For a while we were both silent, unable to find any meaningful words that would make sense in his moment of loss. By his side was a steel tumbler and a plastic water dispenser. On the other shelves built into a wall with peeling paint were his wife's belongings.

Mashkoor Khan retired as an assistant teacher from a government school in Raisen, so named after the eleventh-century fort that towered over the otherwise sleepy town. 'Whatever little I earned as pension, I would hand over to Fatima. She had the command of the house. And of my life.'

The toughest to get through were the nights. Unable to sleep, Mashkoor would toss and turn, and sometimes step out into the lane outside the house and sit on the ledge in the stillness of the darkness, to get some air. One night, he said, a song came to him in his dreams: '*Awaz de kahan hai / Duniya meri jawan hain. Barbad main yahan hu / Abad tu wahan hai.*'

The 1946 song, sung and pictured on Noor Jehan, became a source of solace, a way for Mashkoor to limp from hour to hour, till dawn broke.

A span of just nineteen days had upended all sense of normalcy and well-being for him and his family. After Fatima died, two of Mashkoor's grown-up children, his daughter and son, also succumbed to the illness. Mashkoor was bereft, both as husband and father. But even after three deaths under one roof in quick succession, during the surge of the second wave, the family worried that the official death count would overlook them.

Suhail Mohammed, Mashkoor's son, sat cross-legged on a

string bed in the courtyard of their home, surrounded by a sprawl of paperwork. Letters, hospital discharge slips, prescriptions . . . made up a small mountain. An earthen pot filled with water was placed on the ground beside him. In another side of the open floor, under the shade of a tree, the day's lunch was being prepared in a single pressure cooker.

Suhail traded in fish caught from the Halali river, a tributary of the Betwa river, 40 kilometres from the state capital of Bhopal. His brother Aqeel Ahmad, who died from COVID, used to work at a fuel station. To meet the spiralling costs of medical treatment for his mother and siblings, Suhail finally pawned whatever little jewellery his mother had owned. Like hundreds of thousands of other families, he had a harrowing account of finding an oxygenated bed and moving from government to private hospitals. Now he spent all his energy trying to get official certification of the three deaths. The discharge slip from the Atal Bihari Vajpayee Medical College in Vidisha, the adjoining district where his brother had been hospitalized, did not list COVID as the cause of his death. The hospital's dean told Suhail to attach the results of the RT-PCR test as evidentiary papers at the municipality when he went to register his brother's death. But the local authorities had declined to do so, sending him right back to the hospital. Caught between the two institutions, Suhail worried about how he could approach the government for any of the welfare schemes that had been announced for children who had lost parents to COVID.

Aqeel's three young children were now Suhail's responsibility. They sat on the floor playing with their cousins, wearing Minnie Mouse pink earmuffs, oblivious of the enormity of what had happened. Suhail was still paying interest of ₹1,400 every month on the loan he had taken against the family jewels he had mortgaged. He was terrified about how to manage the additional financial responsibility of his brother's and sister's families.

In Raisen's main bazaar, a short steep flight of stairs led up to a narrow, pan-stained corridor from where you had a direct view of the magnificent fort, rumoured to be haunted. Inside, officials confirmed that on 1 June they received an order from the Economics and Statistics Directorate: it directed registrars to not record the cause in death certificates. That task was to be left to hospitals.

Mashkoor Khan's family wanted official documentation of the three deaths for both emotional and economic reasons. To be counted was about the compact of citizenship. It was also about survival.

The Supreme Court had ordered that compensation be given to the families of those who died from COVID, calling it a 'once in a lifetime pandemic inflicted on the entire world'. The central government initially opposed this, asking whether it was the most 'rational, judicious or optimum' use of resources. Poor households steeped in debt or left without their primary wage earner could not afford to not be counted.

From Madhya Pradesh to Rajasthan, from Gujarat to Tamil Nadu and from Maharashtra to Kerala, in the chaotic aftermath of the pandemic, that most fundamental of questions – how many people died in India from the pandemic – still has no accurate or authentic answer. Worse, there was no institutional impulse to get to the bottom of the inconvenient truth.

Seen from the sky, through a drone's eye, the banks of the Ganga had begun to look like a Jackson Pollock painting – blobs of saffron set haphazardly against the gloomy grey of a large sandy canvas. The radical American painter's drip technique usually involved pouring paint from a can straight on to a backdrop placed horizontally on the floor. From the numbing safety of distance, the pile-up of hundreds of bodies along the denuded riverbanks in Uttar Pradesh and Bihar looked almost similarly artistically organized in their abstract asymmetry and splotches of colour.

The surreal quality of the image notwithstanding, the truth was macabre and all too real. This was the visual manifestation of India's uncounted, unchronicled, undocumented COVID deaths.

Across the world, countries have called for an effort against dehumanization of the dead and to remember that behind every number is a person, a family, a friend, a lover, a child. But this was so much worse. Instead of relegating those who had died to data points – cruel enough in itself – this was a refusal to even count the dead. In other words, those who have died from the virus might not even end up being a statistic.

Deaths have slipped through the official cracks in many countries around the world. Seventeen million people are estimated to have died worldwide when the official numbers count 5 million dead. India's COVID death toll too could be ten times higher than the official count. Put starkly, government figures, as of 21 December, said 478,007 had died from COVID in India; in truth that number could be 4 million. In that case, India would outrank the US to become the country with the highest number of fatalities globally.

We may never be able to precisely say how many of our people have died from COVID, but many Indians have borne witness to the giant difference in the government data and what they saw with their own eyes – images so macabre they will be shadowed by the memories for life. Among them is Jitendra Singh Shunty, conferred in 2021 with the Padma Shri, the fourth highest civilian honour in India. I last met 'Shunty', as he was called, in April 2021 at the Shamshan Ghat in Delhi's Seemapuri area. The cremation ground looked as if someone had dropped a plane-load of petrol on it and then thrown a matchstick in; it was ablaze. Plumes of smoke rose to form a giant grey cover over the entire compound. A mural of Lord Shiva framed the tiled entrance to the cremation site, possibly to lend a moment of serenity to those visiting in sorrow. But that evening he was dwarfed by a row of bodies parked one after the other; there was just no space inside. Strings of marigold placed around a coconut had been left by grieving families in a feeble attempt to lend some dignity and individual emotion to this godawful instance of a mass cremation.

Shunty had been volunteering from the very beginning of the pandemic – helping provide ambulances, food for the poor – and now he was assisting with funeral services. He and his son had both tested positive for COVID in the first year of the pandemic. 'This is a cremation ground where normally you will not see more than ten bodies,' he told me, looking exhausted from lack of sleep. 'In 2020, even at the peak of the surge, I cremated thirty bodies on a single day. But this time, all records have been broken. Just last night we performed the last rites for 122 bodies at one ground. Then I wake up in the morning and see the claim that 350 people have died in all of Delhi! That is outrageous. The actual number is at least twice as high as what we are being told.'

Behind him, his team brought yet more bodies in; they had run short of stretchers now, and some corpses would have to be placed on the floor. The odd jar of ghee, a string of marigold and a half-lit diya were placed in front of some of the bodies. The smoke from the funeral fires made it difficult to breathe. Shunty was agitated. 'The administration expects families to come here with a COVID certificate from the mortuary. But what about all those who are in quarantine at home and die from COVID? My own vans bring such bodies every day. Which account will they go into?'

There are four reasons why undercounting of the dead has been so staggeringly high in India. Those who were not tested for COVID but died during the surge of the first or second wave, whether on the way to the hospital or alone at home, are not counted in the toll. This has happened in large swathes of rural India where there were neither local testing facilities nor enough accessible hospital beds. The bureaucratic process to get a death certificate – some states even passed orders that the cause of death would not be mentioned in the paperwork – left hapless relatives chasing hospitals and administrative officials. Stigma and economic penury played a role in bodies being abandoned without formal registration or even rituals. And deaths that took place as a result of the pandemic – whether from oxygen shortage, mortalities from other illnesses, because the patient could not find a hospital bed, ambulance or doctor, or from lockdown hardships – have not been chronicled as being a consequence of the virus, though they are.

It was towards the end of April in 2021 that Mohit first began to see the bodies. A teenage cowherd tasked with taking cattle out to graze by the riverside in Rautapur, he accidentally bore witness to one of the most cataclysmic events of modern India. At the edge of eastern Uttar Pradesh, in Unnao, Ghongi Rautapur is a sleepy village with fewer than 700 families and 4,000 people. As part of his morning routine, Mohit would walk through the open fields and forest cover out to the banks of the Ganga ghat every day, with half a dozen cows and buffaloes sauntering at a cheerfully lazy pace behind him. It was not unusual for residents from nearby villages to bring in a handful of bodies every few days to be burnt by the riverside on makeshift wooden pyres. But what he was seeing now was dramatically different. Every morning he would arrive by the shore to find fifteen to twenty bodies buried in the sand, some hastily covered with a Ramnami chadar, others unadorned under a mound of mud.

It was on 13 May that I met Mohit, a shy boy with a scraggly frame and a handkerchief tied around his face in lieu of a mask. It was a windswept and stormy morning, and the waters of the usually placid river were lashing angrily against the land boundary. Just by the waves, a body lay burning on a wooden pyre, its flames wrestling with the breeze. There was no one present – no priest chanting a prayer in a soothing, meditative monotone, no son or daughter to gingerly hold an earthen pot and take small, broken steps around the body, no relatives weeping without inhibition in a corner. Whoever had come to perform the last rites of this death had left before they could be seen. The amber glow of the fire cut a lonely and bereft image against the vast expanse of the deserted open field.

There was not just one body, there were more than a hundred buried in the sands around. Mohit pointed to clumps of grass in the mud and said, 'Those are bodies that were buried much earlier.' He then walked us to a corner to show us the two 'fresh' bodies that had been buried in the last twenty-four hours.

Across Uttar Pradesh and Bihar, two states that have crawled at the bottom of the country's Sustainable Development Goals index, villagers call the bodies of the dead *'mitti'*, a word we otherwise understand to mean dust or mud.

At Rautapur, village elders said the surge in bodies, both those being burnt on wood and the those left buried in shallow graves, had coincided with the aftermath of the local elections in the state. The reference was to the escalation in COVID deaths within the government-employed teachers' community that had been forced into poll duty in the month of April.

The next few weeks, I travelled to six different such ghats along the Ganga, covering a distance of several hundred kilometres, in pursuit of unpacking the truth of the mass graves and the staggering distance between the actual and official data on COVID deaths. Journalists tracking COVID deaths have been threatened, abused and vilified as 'vultures' by far-right supporters of the government.

Some of the most important work on India's missing COVID deaths was done not by the national English media, but by local reporters from Hindi newspapers and regional-language publications. *Dainik Bhaskar*, *Sandesh* and *Gujarat Samachar* especially stood out for their shoe-leather reportage. Whether it was staking out at mortuaries or simply counting the number of obituaries in their classified sections and tallying them with the official data, they did sterling public service. But instead of being celebrated, they were abused and vilified, as was I. In July 2021 there were tax raids in multiple cities on the offices of *Dainik Bhaskar*. I was the subject of smear attacks in right-wing-leaning propaganda sites in countries as far as Australia that even dragged my father's death into their innuendo. For some inexplicable reason, the telling of this truth got linked to faux-patriotism. The Western media wasn't showing graves, we were told. But when we would point them towards drone images of mass graves in *The Washington Post* and other publications, the goalpost would be shifted to some other criticism. Most importantly, the families of the dead wanted to speak, wanted to have their tragedies count and very much wanted to resist their invisibilization. Though many of my reports were routinely from both graveyards and cremation grounds, and had been so during both waves, somehow, in 2021, it was the visuals of mass burning pyres that provoked a vicious backlash from some sections.

Of course, in certain circumstances, Hindus have buried their dead instead of burning them – as in the case of infants and young brides, when the practice is to not set fire to the body. Other instances that call for burial, cited by priests, include skin disease and snakebite. But what separated the graves of the Ganga in 2021 from any prior instance was their overwhelming scale. Eyewitness after eyewitness across the cremation grounds I travelled to – Unnao, Kannauj, Kanpur, Kanpur Dehat, Prayagraj – testified to the same truth: in their lifetime they had never seen as many bodies, often abandoned in the cover of night, as they had during the peak of the second wave.

Instead of an official acknowledgement of the crisis or an attempt to reconcile the official death estimates with the real figures, what followed was not just a refusal to acknowledge these mass graves, but an aggressive pushback against anyone who sought to unveil the shroud of deceit and silence thrown over them. For instance, a fictional website, supposedly run out of Australia, was built just to write a column accusing me of feasting off the dead, till Australian journalists called it out for being a fabrication. For tallying the number of pyres at cremation grounds and the burials at graveyards against the official district-wise numbers to show under-reporting, there was an organized campaign to outlaw the publishing of images of cremation and burial grounds.

But while statistics can lie, or at least be miserly with the truth, there is simply no way to hide bodies. Not when they float up the river and wash ashore, literally demanding to be seen, even in the prime minister's constituency.

Sujabad village, a sleepy cluster of homes along the Ganga, is dominated by the Nishad community, the caste group of Uttar Pradesh's boatmen and fisherfolk whose livelihood is tied to the river. In early May, Phoolchand Baba, an elderly local resident, lithe and agile for his years, his lungi wrapped efficiently around his lean frame, strode purposefully over the mud and gravel to point out the fresh mounds that had just been dug up. An empty packet of salt fluttered in the wind just above a small crater in the ground. A group of fishermen were waist deep in the river water just behind us; others sat on their haunches, their lungis tucked into their waists, looking out at what the river may wash up next. Seven bodies, those of men and women both, had floated ashore that week, in a half-decomposed condition. Villagers helped local authorities dig up resting places for them. The salt was to eliminate the smell that would otherwise draw dogs and other animals to the corpses. '*Bodies Gangaji se aayee*,' (The bodies came from the Ganga) said Phoolchand, using the honorific for Hinduism's most revered river.

The Ganga traverses 2,500 kilometres from its origin in the Himalayas all the way to the Bay of Bengal. Legend has it that she was lowered on to earth by Shiva's hair, a journey that spanned 1,000 years. Devout Hindus personify the river as a goddess and attribute to her powers to cleanse them of their sins.

But now the Ganga was regurgitating corpses.

'Perhaps they came from the houses across the river,' said Phoolchand, pointing to a settlement in the distance. The bodies had obviously been abandoned, a pattern that would repeat itself with insidious regularity through the two months of the second wave. As a train chugged along the 'double decker' bridge over Varanasi's Rajghat, so called because it was a two-tier structure that allowed vehicles on one level and a rail track on the other,

Phoolchand was excited to share that he'd had the chance to see the prime minister in flesh and blood just a couple of years ago. The adjoining village of Domri had been adopted by Modi under the model village scheme for parliamentarians. A few days later Modi fought back tears as he addressed the health workers of Varanasi.

But even when confronted with the evidence of mass graves, the government continued to contest the overwhelming evidence of massive under-reporting of COVID deaths. Unless there is a countrywide audit and a sincere effort to count every fatality, we will never know how many hundreds of thousands of more Indians have died than we know or have been told have. Epidemiologists compute this by a method called excess mortality, which basically factors deaths from all causes, COVID and non-COVID, in a fixed time frame, and compares that figure to the average death count in the corresponding period of previous years. These 'extra' or excess deaths are one scientific clue as to how many more people are dying than usual in a pandemic. While not all of these deaths will be from COVID – in fact, a separate study will have to be conducted on how many died from non-COVID infectious diseases simply because of their inability to access healthcare – it is reasonable to assume that at least half are. The mismatch is staggering. Madhya Pradesh's excess deaths were 42 times the reported COVID deaths; Andhra Pradesh recorded 34 times excess deaths, and Kerala 1.6 times its official COVID death toll. By the second week of May, modellers argued that over a million Indians had already died from COVID. The official data was skewed by a factor of anywhere between 5 and 7. In the same month, Uttar Pradesh, which had presented the most dramatic visual manifestation of this under-reporting, was congratulated for being a 'model state'.

There was no need for calculators, Excel sheets, columns or models if you travelled along the Ganga and made the effort to reach the absolute peripheries of major towns. Many of these areas were remote, not easily accessible by road and tough to navigate on foot because of the thick layers of sticky sand and loose stones on the banks. In Kanpur, the industrial town known for leather shoes and cotton mills, bodies piled up at two different focal points. The only way to get to the ghats under the district's newly minted flyovers was to find an opening in the rocky ravine, hop on to the back of a motorcycle and ride through the trenches. We were two hours away from the city and there was no one to be seen for miles, except a solitary shopkeeper frying samosas for passing truckers in a dimly lit thatched hut. Over the period of a fortnight, he had personally seen anywhere between 100 and 150 bodies brought to the grounds every day. The path to the ghat was not car friendly. The day we visited we were lucky enough to meet two local photographers and persuade them to take me along on their bike. And there, in the shadows of conical electricity towers that reached for the sky, were hundreds of bodies scattered all around, between clumps of grass and pebbles, the concave pits pointing to the human beings buried just below. There were some remnants of life – a solitary leather slipper, a steel tumbler, a bottle of half-used medicinal syrup – in the deserted landscape. We discovered there were two kinds of farewells at the ghats. One, a regular cremation, where the family accompanied the body, often in a tractor that was also the hearse, waited for the wood to turn to ash, said their prayers and left. And the other was the hastily discarded goodbye, either in the river or at its flanks.

In Prayagraj, which most Indians knew better as Allahabad – so named by the emperor Akbar – till Adityanath renamed it, the local pandit warned of an impending public health disaster as we waded through open drains and past cows and dogs. The bodies that had been brought recently were buried closer to the river. There was a single coconut left by the side of one, and a marigold garland strung around another. Four small pillars, like the corners of a poster bed, made from bamboo thickets, marked the boundaries of a few. Mishraji, the pandit, believed there were two reasons for the deluge of abandoned corpses – the social stigma around COVID and the extreme poverty of the families the dead came from, made worse by fifteen months of lockdowns, which made a wood pyre unaffordable for many. As bare-chested boys frolicked in the water behind us, enviably oblivious that they were surrounded by gigantic tragedy, Mishraji described the scenes that he had witnessed this year that he had never seen in all his years. 'Seventy–eighty bodies were being left every day, *poora mela laga hua tha.*' He warned that when the monsoons came the shallow graves would be wrenched open by the force of the water and the bodies would flow back into the river. '*Bimari ka ghar ban jayega.*' (This will become a house of disease.)

At Kannauj and Nanamau ghats, witnesses I met were united on one thing: what was unfolding was unprecedented in scale. At the sprawling grounds of Mehndi Ghat, the earth was swollen with bodies in the hundreds. In the distance, the plastic blue of a PPE suit broke the sea of orange formed by the shrouds. The embankment was swarming with people who had arrived from far-flung villages in tractors filled beyond carrying capacity. These were the 'normal' funerals, staggering for the massive number of fires lit all along the water. But just a footstep behind were the bodies that had no name, no address and no heartbroken father or mother who might collapse on their knees in unspeakable grief by the grave of their son or daughter. Raj Narain, an employee at the cremation ground, told me: 'In my twelve years here I have never seen what I see now. If earlier, twenty to fifty bodies came in a day, that number has doubled now.'

By now I had personally counted more than 500 corpses across the five river towns I had reported from. From the banks of Mehndi Ghat I took a boat down the Ganga, making a 30-kilometre journey downstream to the next major funeral site. The boat was powered by a do-it-yourself motor that was ignited by the pulling of a string. We sailed to the sound of its loud metallic croak till the shoreline could no longer be seen. In deeper waters, Subhash, the boatman, switched off the motor and the boat's buoyancy moved it gently over the muddy, greenish-blue parts of the river. In the distance buffaloes and stray dogs waded into the water. Accompanied by Mayank, a young boy who maintained the register of entries at the grounds, we went past tiny rural settlements and saw bodies being burnt out in the open, with mostly men standing around, stoic and wordless, dressed in crisp white kurtas and turbans. In the four weeks that coincided with the peak of the second wave, Mayank said he had seen approximately 1,500 bodies at the ghat. Families were coming from faraway towns too because space had run out at local cremation grounds. He too believed fear and stigma were driving the mass abandonment of bodies. Most of these people came when the sun went down and the twilight provided cover for stealth. Subhash, whose family plied seven boats up and down the river ferrying passengers, said this month he had shut operations. In his thirty-two years of being a boatman he had 'never seen so many bodies. *Mujhe ghabrahat hone lagee.* (I started feeling anxious.) One body would barely be buried or burnt and another one would arrive. I felt like running away to a place where I did not have to see another human body ever again.'

I asked Subhash if he had been tested for COVID. But there were no testing facilities in his village. 'If I could get one, why wouldn't I want one.'

This was another big reason why hundreds of thousands of deaths did not make it to the official registry. In villages across India, from Tamil Nadu in the south to Madhya Pradesh in the west, people were dying at home before they could get an RT-PCR test or access a hospital. They had all the symptoms of COVID, including fever and difficulty in breathing, but were never tabulated because they were never officially diagnosed.

In the Chennasandiram panchayat of Hosur, Jaykumar Reddy, the president of a cluster of seven villages, told me there was no operational primary health centre in his area. By now, twenty deaths had taken place over just four weeks in hutments where most people were small farmers. The deaths had added to the anxiety about making a trip to the city in an attempt to find a hospital that would run a COVID test. 'Give us vaccines, give us testing kits,' implored Reddy. 'The villagers cannot go to the city. The hospital must come to us.'

The official files may not tell you the truth about how many Indians have died in the pandemic. But they do give you a reasonable glimpse into a broken, neglected rural healthcare system. The Economic Survey (2019–20) shows that India's primary healthcare network needs 21,340 specialist doctors; the country is short by 17,549. Rural India has 3.2 government beds for every 10,000 people; states like Uttar Pradesh, Rajasthan and Jharkhand have even lower numbers. Maharashtra, the state which had the highest number of COVID cases in the country, had 2 beds for every 10,000 citizens, and Bihar brings up the rear at 0.6.

In Basi village, in western Uttar Pradesh, just two hours

from the national capital, where winding roads weave their way through lush sugarcane fields, the locals said nearly every home had someone with a fever in the nearly 5,000-strong community. Rajesh, a village elder, told us that thirty-five villagers had died in less than a month, some of them men in their twenties. He had written many letters to the local administration, but no intervention had come. When we went to the local health centre, it was locked, and creepers were growing over the gates. No one had been by in several months. The onset of fever in the village was not followed by a COVID test; instead, local doctors would typically diagnose it as typhoid or pneumonia. By the time a hospital was looked for it was already too late. This could mean entire families wiped out without being listed in the government database.

In Praveen Kumar's house, his children knelt before two photographs placed by a clutch of roses on the stone floor of their courtyard. One was the picture of Kanwar Sain Singh, fifty-nine, their grandfather, and the other was his son, their uncle Parvender, who was only thirty-one years old. The day we met them, the *havan* prayers to bid farewell to both were still being read. Incense filled the small room where Praveen took out the family album, ran a cloth over its dusty cover and spoke of how his brother had died within a day of his father's demise. His father had never been tested for COVID; till guidelines were changed a hospital admission was not possible without such a test. By the time Praveen was able to get him to a hospital, he was gasping for breath. The doctors in the district hospital of Baghpat placed him on oxygen, but thirty minutes later he was dead. However, because he had never had a test done, he would never be listed or counted in the government database.

The other reason for the systemic invisibilization of India's

COVID deaths is the staggering number of people who died on the streets, in ambulances, in hospital corridors, simply looking for a bed that they were never fortunate enough to find, especially during the second surge.

Some travelled hundreds of kilometres before dying on the way. When Rudresh, a small-time painter in Bengaluru, tested positive for COVID and could not find a hospital with a free bed anywhere in his city of work, his sister suggested he return home to his village in Tamil Nadu, an hour's drive across the state border. Initially Rudresh was treated for his fever at the local hospital. But when his oxygen levels started to dip the doctors advised that he upgrade to an ICU bed. His two teenage daughters and sisters jumped on to the back of an ambulance with him. So began their hunt across three cities of Karnataka and Tamil Nadu, till they ended up back in Bengaluru where they had started. As they sat outside a private hospital waiting for 'an OTP alert' on their phones from the centralized system, Rudresh died. Because he did not die inside a COVID ward of a hospital he will never be counted among the dead.

And so it was, in city after city.

Bhopal's JP Nagar colony is across the street from what was once the Union Carbide factory. Even today you can see the giant drums in the compound of the now-shut gas company from the very entrance to the neighbourhood. The one-room tenements are tiny, with almost no walls separating one from the other, and the homes are arranged around open drainpipes and serpentine alleys. Stray dogs sleep in the scorching summer sun. Some homes have pet parrots in cages strung from a rope tied to their terraces. In screeching falsetto voices, the birds mimic the sounds and speech of visitors – mostly journalists and social workers who annually revisit the colossal tragedy that took place in this corner of the city. In December 1984, methyl isocyanate, 500 times more poisonous than cyanide, leaked from the Union Carbide premises and killed 5,000 people in a single day. JP Nagar was ravaged. Among them were the parents of Vikas Chauhan, an autorickshaw driver. The family must have believed that destiny's preordained quota of tragedy for them had been exhausted. But the day Vikas fell ill, his wife Jyoti packed him into the rickshaw he rode, asked a neighbour to take control of the wheel and went all across the city in search of help. She watched him struggle to breathe, hitting the air with his hands as his oxygen levels sank. They spent five hours on the road and were turned away from six hospitals before they returned home in resignation and despair. Vikas died at the doorway of the steep staircase leading to his house. But again, he will not be listed as one of India's COVID dead.

In the lane adjacent to Jyoti's is Kiran Tomar's house. She whispered to us to speak to her outside; she did not want her husband, a terminally ill cancer patient, to hear our conversation. A soft-spoken woman, she was draped in a yellow sari that she had taken over her head. Kiran said there was no money now to place food on the table. Her two sons died within a week of each other, in a matter of seven days; one has been listed as a COVID death, the other remains undocumented. The elder son was the first to go. Manoj Tomar, forty-one, was diagnosed by the local clinic to have typhoid or what commonly went by the name of *motijhara* in Hindi. The doctor prescribed a bunch of medicines and never recommended a test for COVID. A few days later, a second medical opinion urged a COVID test. Manoj, whose condition had worsened, started looking for help, but it was too late and he died before he could be tested. His brother died from COVID a week later. Kiran hopes that when she finally gets his death certificate it will list a cause of death that will entitle them to compensation.

In state after state, town after town, we tailed families that spent hours outside dingy municipal corporations in the hope of being formally recognized as having lost their loved ones to COVID by the administration. Most families, lower-income as well as middle-class ones, took loans, mortgaged jewellery or sold land to pay the hefty hospital bills at private facilities. Many were asked to arrange for injections like remdesivir and tocilizumab on their own. They had to pay for these drugs in cash in the black market so that even if they were insured they could not claim compensation. Earning members have died in hundreds of thousands of homes. Compensation is not just a moral principle; it is a financial imperative.

'*Dard hee dard.*' (An endless cycle of pain.) That's how Ramavatar Singh, a block-print worker in Jaipur, Rajasthan, summed up how he felt after he lost his wife Santosh Devi to COVID. She was young, only thirty-five, a striking-looking woman in the photographs he shares with us, dressed in a monochromatic red kurta salwar, with maroon lipstick to match. They had two small children, a boy and a girl, just twelve and eight years old. They sat on upturned Dalda cans by his side at a streetside tea shop across the road from his factory, silent and scared. 'I cannot describe my pain; I have lost my life partner. I did everything I could to save her.'

Ramavatar took a loan of ₹300,000 from his factory owner to get his wife treated at a private hospital. Since she died, he told me, he had to make three trips to the hospital just to get the documents for discharge. When the hospital finally handed him the papers he asked why the release form did not mention COVID. '*Bas, aise hee bante hai, bhaiyya, le jao, or jao.*' (That is how these papers are made. Just take them and go.)

Ramavatar worried about being able to manage as a single father. 'If there is some welfare scheme for my children, I won't even be able to help them,' he said, absolutely crestfallen. 'This is after my wife spent twelve days in a hospital being treated for COVID.' Finally, after multiple trips to the hospital and to government offices, Ramavatar Singh was able to procure a death certificate. But it did not list COVID as the cause of death.

It would have been no consolation to Ramavatar Singh, but in Ratan Sagar Colony, a somewhat more upscale neighbourhood of Jaipur, Shrichand, a government employee who issues death certificates, could not get one for his wife either. He was now urging his department to change the rules.

With or without a piece of paper, the dead are speaking from their graves. Lying alongside the river most revered by Indians, they are determined to have their stories told.

And so, it shouldn't surprise us that there was a half-baked attempt to silence them.

It was towards the end of May when the police in Prayagraj stood around the dry riverbanks officiously and ordered that the saffron shrouds be taken off the bodies that had piled up one after the other, like a car crash on a major highway. Poor labourers, without any protective gear, were enlisted to wade into the sticky sand to erase the last bit of empirical evidence of uncounted COVID deaths. When there was outrage, a probe was ordered into how and why this had happened.

But the images and the truth could not remain unseen.

And in July 2021, when the monsoon hit a parched land, it opened up the shallow graves revealing the corpses that lay just beneath, nudging them back into the river from where they had washed ashore, demanding to be counted.

The chroniclers and eyewitnesses of the COVID pandemic have been its pallbearers, the volunteers who cremated and buried bodies when no one else would. The stigma around handling a body was much more pointed during the first wave, when corpses were abandoned in hospital mortuaries. Families were not willing to step near their own. But during the second wave too, abandoned bodies were not unusual. The essential humanism of the Indian people is reflected in the courage and compassion of those who stepped forward to transcend a toxic television-induced environment of religious hatred.

11

The COVID Pallbearers

Funerals for Lonely Humans

If ever there were four words that captured the emotional deprivation, social isolation and institutional breakdown of the pandemic years, here they were.

The words were scrawled in bright blood-red across the side of a white van that was now a repurposed ambulance, that at a pinch also doubled up as a hearse.

The van was always left in first gear and ready to go. In May 2020, it was parked in the open space in the front side of the one-room office of Ekta Trust, next to a stockpile of wooden logs (firewood for cremations) and right across the street from Surat's main church.

Abdul Rehman Malbari, a sprightly middle-aged man with a youthful restlessness, was getting ready to jump into the front seat and drive to the civil hospital. The death was of a Hindu woman. From the hospital he would have to drive with the hearse to a cremation site.

His premises were tiny. A bare table and chair were placed in a room that was as narrow as a phone booth. A slightly bigger adjacent room was chock-a-block with ceremonial material haphazardly organized in colourful, untidy piles that rose from floor to ceiling. There were casket sheets and prayer mats for Muslim burials, but also Gangajal and ghee for Hindu cremations. Malbari performed both, making sure to take a photograph of the rituals to share with families later, so relatives could be reassured that those they loved had been sent off with dignity. Countless others were simply left to die, at the gates of graveyards and crematoriums or inside hospital wards.

In the early months of the pandemic there was still little known about the airborne spread of the virus. The belief was that mere touch and proximity to infected surfaces could be lethal. WHO guidelines, as well as government guidelines, had an extremely strict protocol for the handling of bodies. Bathing and embalming of corpses were banned, as were touching, holding and kissing them. The strict regimen, prolonged lockdown, poverty and prejudice (gigantic stigma powered by bad science and fake news about how COVID could be contracted made it worse) led many families to abandon their own who died.

'Our job is not just to conduct the rituals, we also make sure that we meet the family thereafter and assure them that everything was done according to belief,' Malbari said. He wore a blue flak jacket emblazoned with 'Ekta' in gold over his plain kurta. He expounded at length over the distinction in the rituals; the *mitti* he carried to disperse over the graves, the sacred water he kept to sprinkle over the pyres.

Malbari, who had set up his small volunteer force after the Gujarat earthquake in 2001, had long made it his mission to provide dignity in death to those who had remained unloved in life. But nothing he had done in the aftermath of limited natural calamities – in peacetime his work was limited to the burial of the body of a beggar or a homeless man who would die unmourned on the streets – had prepared him for this.

With almost no one willing to handle bodies, not even those of their own parents, lovers or siblings, the city's municipal corporation had tasked Malbari with the job.

That he was a Muslim, now immersed in all the Hindu rituals of last rites, right from slokas to sandalwood, did not strike him as the least bit comment-worthy.

'I am more scared of the living than the dead. The bodies – before they are Hindu or Muslim – they are human.'

At any other time, this would have been a truism, a self-evident do-gooder statement that may have even been overlooked for its obvious good manners.

But Indian public discourse had already been coarsened by a communal, poisonous conversation around the role of the Tablighi Jamaat, an orthodox Sunni sect, as a super-spreader. The proselytizing organization, which urged believers to return to Islam as practised in the age of the Prophet, was spread across eighty countries with its *markaz* or centre in Delhi. In early March 2020, roughly ten days before India was officially locked down, a religious congregation was organized in the capital's Nizamuddin area, a Muslim-dominated neighbourhood made up of untidy, byzantine lanes where fourteenth-century domes built from red sandstone and inlaid marble shared space with overcrowded slums, pavement dwellers and child beggars. An advisory from the Delhi government had warned against gatherings of more than 200 people but did not specifically ban religious events. Hundreds of foreigners had also entered India from COVID hotspots like Indonesia and Malaysia to attend the congregation held between 13 and 15 March. A few thousand pilgrims attended the event. Thereafter, the oblivious

Tablighis fanned out in different directions of India, carrying the virus with them. It was only after the first COVID case was traced back to the Tablighis in Tamil Nadu that the Centre sounded the alarm across states and a massive contact-tracing programme started.

That the organization of a mass event in the middle of a pandemic was criminally negligent was never in dispute. But there were lapses all around. Malaysia and Indonesia had already emerged as COVID flashpoints in Southeast Asia, and there too a gathering of the Tablighi Jamaat at a mosque on 28 February had led to a sharp spike in cases. And yet, in the first three months of the year, more than 2,000 foreigners were able to enter the country without any screening or restrictions. By the end of March more than 800 of them had dispersed to different destinations across India.

As the remaining Tablighis were finally evacuated in the busloads, television networks began smearing the entire Muslim community in language that normalized religious hatred. Phrases like 'Corona jihad' were used to suggest a wilful spread of the virus. Prime-time anchors referenced visual graphics on rising cases depicting the numbers against silhouettes of men in skullcaps. The hashtag #CoronaJihad was used over 300,000 times and was seen by 165 million people in less than a week.[28] There were other religious communities that were on pilgrimages when the lockdown was announced by the prime minister – Sikhs at the gurudwara in Nanded in Maharashtra, Hindus at Vaishno Devi in Jammu – but the language used for them in mainstream media was very different. When they were brought back to their states, it was a homecoming. By contrast, multiple headlines spoke of the Tablighis as having been 'hiding' in mosques across the country.

The pandemic reinforced prejudices, both obvious and latent. It did so not just in India, where differences of class, gender and religion were magnified in an almost macabre, bare-boned way; but also in societies globally, including America, where Trump's characterization of the virus as 'Chinese' led to a spate of attacks on Asian Americans.

In India, paradoxically, in a Dickensian besting and worsting of times, the breakdown of social and community structures ran parallel to extraordinary displays of courage and compassion.

And nowhere was this more evident than in the stories of those who stepped up to be the pallbearers of COVID.

It was a job no one else was ready to do.

In the early months of the pandemic, Dr Kalpana Baliwant, an official with the Pune city corporation, broke down in tears at the Rahat Bagh Kabristan as she sought the help of a group of volunteers in the otherwise deserted burial grounds. Shrubs and trees formed a gentle canopy over freshly dug mounds of graves. The sun's rays hit at sharp perpendicular angles, forming a hard shadow over a lone aluminium stretcher, normally used to ferry the dead on their last mile. Birds chirped softly in the distance. There were not even any grieving relatives or people milling around, offering comforting hugs or a glass of water to a distraught wife or brother, in a country where an entire village usually turns up to say goodbye.

Baliwant said people were leaving their family members to die outside hospitals, sometimes even out on the streets. In other instances, relatives were refusing to even own their dead. Two bodies lay outside the city's civil hospital for several days till the police had to be deployed to trace who they were. Official staff at government-run funeral sites were refusing to show up. And even the drivers of the ambulance hearses refused to drive with a COVID body at the back. Such was the fear of the unknown. 'I have seen the worst of humanity,' Baliwant said,

The COVID pallbearers – Hindu, Muslim, Sikh and Christian – were the handymen tasked to repair and reassemble the broken bits of our humanity. Nearly all were poor or of modest means. Many had spent years at the very bottom of the caste or economic ladder, socially discriminated against, even though it is in their hands that we place the bodies of those who have our hearts. They are the gravediggers, the body washers, the corpse burners and the furnace cleaners, the conduit between the end of this life and whatever lies on the other side.

'The virus does not distinguish between Hindu and Muslim,' said Jagdish Paswan, a mortuary worker at Indore's private Aurobindo Medical College. Flanked by Golu, Sohanlal and Lakhan, all Hindus, these were the men who buried the bodies of the Muslim patients who died at the hospital. Dressed in maroon scrubs and masks, they stood with both pride and purpose, like soldiers stationed at the borderline. 'Families are not ready to touch the bodies, so we do it for them,' said Jagdish, barely flinching as a corpse wrapped like a mummy from head to toe was wheeled in on a stretcher as we spoke. Fourteen per cent of Indore's population is Muslim, but as Golu asked me: 'What does religion have to do with anything, isn't this about humanity?' His words provoked a spontaneous applause from those who were listening to our conversation – security guards, sweepers, technical staff. What may have sounded like homilies and platitudes in peacetime had acquired an urgent moral force in a mass-media-generated environment of hate.

At the Jadeed Qabristan, a haven of quiet tucked away behind the traffic snarls of ITO in Delhi, one of the busiest road junctions in the world, Mohammed Shamim was forced to pull at gravel and stones with his bare hands after the men who steered the bulldozers and drove the heavy JCB excavators refused to show up at work. In its ninety-seven-year history, this sprawling, leafy haven of stillness had never run short of space. But now Shamim, a towering, tall man who was lean as a twig and wore a baseball cap over his long kurta and short pyjamas, had to cut through brambles and bushes to clear more space for graves. Walking through what was 'once a jungle', he pointed to his clothes, the rough and tumble, mismatched cottons on his skin. 'We touch the bodies that no one else is willing to keep. But our PPE kits have run out. We have no gloves, no protective gear.' The twenty kits given to him by the local municipal authorities right at the beginning of the pandemic had been used, reused (though strictly not meant to be) and thrown away. 'But I still have to do this job. If I don't, who will?' Between March and June of 2020, Shamim buried 240 bodies himself, both COVID and suspected COVID. He finally found one man, Sher Singh, who agreed to operate the JCB machine. Shamim motioned in the direction of a sunny yellow truck that stood in the distance, its jaw buckets and arms lined with fresh blobs of soil. 'Sheru,' he called out, in convivial familiarity, 'come here for a second.'

Sheru came sprinting towards us, a short, sprightly man who was no taller than Shamim's shoulder. He was wearing a tomato-red Carlsberg T-shirt, hand-me-down black trackpants and a big smile. Of all the machine operators Shamim had reached out to, only Sheru, a Hindu, had agreed to take on the job of running the hydraulic machine through the rocks and stones to make way for the bodies of Muslims who were dying from COVID. 'It's *pagalpan*,' Sheru said, 'to do Hindu-Muslim politics in the middle of a pandemic. Shamim and I – we are brothers.'

As COVID became less mysterious and science progressed

enough for us to know that the mere touching of common surfaces was not how the virus spread – the transmission was swiftest from people breathing the same air in closed spaces – the associated stigma gradually reduced, at least in India's cities. But the stigma against those who performed the public service of funerals and burials never diminished.

. . . Not even in the months when they were among the most sought-after men.

Varanasi's ghats, where believers bring their dead in search of salvation, even have their own raja. The 'king' of the Dom community is the leader of the Dalit sub-caste that has historically been the keeper of the sacred flame – the pyres are lit with this flame and never a matchstick – at the Raja Harishchandra and Manikarnika funeral grounds by the Ganga. In 2019, this 'chief cremator' was one the four nominees who proposed the name of Narendra Modi as candidate from the constituency in 2014. But the Doms, much sought after in moments of bereavement, are still reviled by the living. Barred from temples and weddings, they have lived a life of continued social exclusion despite the occasional media spotlight.

Over two consecutive summers, as space shrank at the riverbanks and bodies stacked up like a macabre mountain of pending laundry, cremation grounds became battlefields. There was jostling for space, shouting over the exorbitant cost of wood and continuing uncertainty and fear over whether it was safe to be proximate to the bodies of those who had died.

The job of preparing the bodies for the last rites was that of the body washers of Varanasi. They said they were in their early twenties, but some of them were clearly still teenagers. They received the bodies at small, ramshackle outposts before they were taken to the pyres for burning. In the alleyways of India's most sacred city, once described by Mark Twain as 'older than history, older than legend, older than tradition', these young men would bathe and embalm the corpses before they were taken to the banks of the Ganga for their final send-off. While others associated with the dead – ambulance drivers, grieving relatives, government officials – came to the grounds covered in head-to-toe sheaths of white and blue plastic, these young men stood out in the crowd, milling about casually and dressed carelessly in shorts and shirts. While a couple of them wore simple disposable masks, most wore an oversized cotton gamcha wrapped across their nose and mouth, the gamchas' spare length hanging loosely over their chins. They worked in shifts, ten to a group, covering all twenty-four hours of the day, since cremations were running through the night. On the ground behind them a body was being draped with marigolds before it would be carried on their shoulders, down the steep stone steps right by the river.

Like many other ancient traditions, Varanasi's body washers were part of an age-old informal economy that had sprung up around the ghats. Today, a harassed, grieving relative was shouting at them and accusing them of charging too much money. Deepak, a gangly lad wearing only a sleeveless vest, who appeared to be the self-appointed leader of this disparate group, turned around and said, 'We also have to feed our families, we are risking our lives doing this every day, doing what no one else is ready to do.' No one had thought to distribute proper masks to these boys who came into daily, relentless contact with COVID corpses. Deepak shrugged off the absence of PPE kits. In any case, he explained, they would 'suffocate and die' if they had to be draped in sheaths in the summer sun, considering their day was spent around fires and furnaces. 'That's all right, we take the risk with our eyes open. But has anyone stopped to notice that the wealthiest Indians are unwilling to come near their dead, they stand a few feet away and throw flowers at the body. It's left to us to handle everything at great risk to our lives. And we are poor people. We help those who come through government channels for free.'

We made our way past stockpiles of wooden logs spilling on to the narrow road that led to the pyres. 'In Hindu dharma, the most important thing when someone dies is to give the *arthi* a *kandha*,' Deepak said, talking of the traditional shoulder offered to the deceased before the flames consume the body, conventionally the duty of the men in the family. 'Families aren't ready to touch the people they claim to love; we do it, and they still judge us, vilify us. What we are doing is public service.'

Across India, local government bodies, collapsing under the weight of the calamity, were falling back on volunteers and informally organized groups like Varanasi's body washers. But that came with its own economic and social insecurity. 'Right now there is COVID, so we are in demand. When this pandemic ends, who will even remember us? They will just kick us and throw us out here. Where will we go then?' asked another lad from within the group.

All of a sudden, Deepak interrupted and said, 'Actually, you should know, my real name is Om Yadav. I made up this fictional name so that no one in my neighbourhood recognizes me and what I do. My reputation is *badnaam*, ruined.' Deepak, who was actually Om, explained that handling the dead always triggered some degree of discrimination, but ever since he started washing the bodies of those who died in the pandemic, he had become an 'untouchable'. People would wave him out of shops, neighbours would ask him to keep his distance, and even relatives at home weren't ready to sit down and eat in the same room as he.

Across cities and religious communities there were mirror images of this phenomenon.

In the walled city of Hyderabad, one house stood out for the murals on its wall. A riot of fluorescent colours had been used to paint tigers prowling in the jungle, trees laden with fruits, flowers in bloom and all kinds of potted plants. At the garish green door of the entrance two children stood giggling over a shared secret joke. It looked almost like an Indian version of a Hansel and Gretel candy house imagined from a comic book. But step inside and the vibrant facade made way for a crumbling interior of an old house organized haphazardly around an open courtyard. The food for that evening's meal – rice with small bits of mutton – was being cooked over a charcoal fire, out in the open, in an aluminium utensil the size of a bucket. Next to it was a cauldron of muddy water for washing both vessels and vegetables. Seventy members of one extended clan, known locally as the Ghasals within the city's Muslim community, lived in this dilapidated structure. A toddler no older than three had a broom in his hand and was running over the tiled courtyard with it. Others sat cross-legged on the cool floor, next to steel trunks and plastic chairs piled up with half-folded clothes and sheets. A clothes line with wet clothes stretched from one end of the house to the other, hanging precariously like a threat over a couple of two-wheelers. The back door of the house opened up to a graveyard that extended for a few miles.

Like the others in the family, Safiya Begum had spent years bathing and preparing the corpses of Muslim women before they were buried. She had continued to do this during the pandemic, till she tested positive after washing the body of an elderly Muslim woman in her eighties who had been confirmed to have died from COVID. But when Safiya was called to conduct the last rituals, she had no idea that she was handling a virus-infected corpse. Safiya was somewhat of a pariah in the neighbourhood now, but as a mother to four she worried about how to make ends meet if she and her relatives halted their work temporarily. Each body they washed helped the family earn ₹500.

Mohammed Omar, the patriarch of the community, proudly pulled out an identity card. 'Dead Body washer,' it said, listing his blood group and other sundry details. It had been issued to him by the '*Kafan* shop' of the Jama Masjid of Afzal Gunj, the local mosque. Kafan, the Urdu word for coffin shroud, is the professional hallmark of this family. Omar showed us his credentials in the same way a doctor might his medical degree; there was the workman's pride in his craft and service. He even had government certification, which he displayed as it was the ultimate endorsement of his traditional work. But now he and his community were living an existential crisis: on the one hand was the spectre of possible death if they continued to work, and on the other potential starvation.

That among both Hindus and Muslims an insidious social hierarchy relegated some caste groups and sects to handle the dead – leaving them at the receiving end of lifelong discrimination – was barely remarked upon. It was just one of the many inequities COVID stripped the veil off, forcing us to take notice.

The truly extraordinary chronicles of compassion were written by those whose income or duty was not tied to looking after the dead.

In Bengaluru, India's information technology hub, Raghu Prasad Rao was one of the cogs who spun the mighty wheel of India's $180 billion BPO industry. A short flight of stairs led up to a sparsely furnished one-bedroom apartment, where Rao was sitting cross-legged with his daughter on the bed, encouraging her to paint and colour. Manushree, nine, was still unaware that her mother, Swarnalata, a teacher, who was pregnant with her second baby, had died from COVID at thirty-five. The baby she had been carrying had to be aborted as doctors struggled to save her life. Raghu, emotionally reticent and not given to giant displays of emotion, did not have the heart to tell the truth to his daughter just yet. Soft fairy lights were strung over a mirror, giving Manushree's room a pink glow as the daylight mingled with the reflected glow of the electric bulbs. A portrait of Lord Krishna, cheeky, irreverent, full of joy, stared down at the young girl. A golden hair band held back Manushree's short bob. She leaned over her book somewhat mechanically, filling the tortoise stencil with a mix of yellow and blue. 'I want to be a doctor when I'm older,' said Manushree, her wistful eyes lighting up briefly at the thought of returning to school. A pair of orange-coloured toy stethoscopes framed the wall. 'I wanted to be one even before COVID,' she declared, with a wan smile.

Raghu shushed us out of the room and up to the terrace so we could speak more freely. 'I have told my daughter her mother has gone to meet Goddess Durga, that they are together and they are fighting COVID,' he said, falling silent for a few seconds, choking with tears as he recounted the horror of moving his wife across three different hospitals. Five days before Swarnalata lost her battle to COVID, her still-to-be-born daughter had a cardiac arrest. Doctors had to operate to remove the body of the baby from the womb. The first hospital Swarnalata was admitted to, a government-run medical centre, had no oxygen bed. The second, a private hospital, had no paediatric ICU or operation theatre available. Finally, it was at the third that both mother and child died. Rao, also ill with COVID, had to stay at home through it all, borrowing money from friends and family and dispatching it to the three hospitals whenever he could. 'I feel no anger, I just feel helpless. What is the use of anger?'

Swarnalata's death broke Raghu's spirit. He could not bring himself to bury his six-month-old. Babies are not cremated in the Hindu tradition because of the belief that they are too young, pure and innocent to need release from the karmic cycle of birth and rebirth. Raghu adjusted his mask, moved his spectacles up the bridge of his nose and fought back tears. 'Actually, I just did not have the courage, I did not have the strength.'

It is then that Raghu called Ibrahim Akram, a volunteer with a group called Mercy Angels. Akram, a restaurateur who owns a Chinese fast-food chain called Beijing Bites, had begun his public service in the pandemic by throwing his kitchen open to a group of activists with 'United Sikhs', who created freshly cooked packed meals for healthcare workers. As the pandemic got worse and the needs mounted, Akram sold a 1952 vintage Fiat car he owned to raise more funds. Over time, he realized that while many were willing to send food and clothes for the poor and needy and for those who were serving at the front line, the real gap was at cremation grounds, mortuaries and graveyards.

'He took my daughter and promised me he would bury her with all the sacred rituals,' said Raghu, overwhelmed by the memories – of both what Akram did for his family and that he could not be there himself. 'I gave my unborn baby to Ibrahim. He gave her dignity.'

There's a photograph that captures that moment. Ibrahim, bent over mud that is still loose and scattered, placing in a cavity the size of a small box an infant wrapped in yellow cloth that is as bright as the shade of the sun. Ibrahim is haunted by the image. 'Raghu told me, don't burn my baby, bury her, whether you do that in a Muslim burial ground or a Hindu funeral site, I don't care, just don't burn her.'

Ibrahim Akram had nowhere to take the child's corpse immediately. That evening he placed her in the freezer of a Muslim burial ground. The next morning, he buried her at a Hindu crematorium, as her father had wished. Five days later, he helped the family cremate Swarnalata.

Raghu showed us a video from the school where Swarnalata taught. She and a Muslim colleague perform a small skit for the students in which they speak about the festivals of Vara Mahalakshmi and Bakr Eid. They speak of pluralism and celebrating the faith and practices of the other.

'Ibrahim is my brother now,' said Raghu. 'He is my family. And Manushree will be brought up on those values.'

The physical closure of schools in India during the two years of the pandemic has costs that are still being understood and studied. Millions of children have been pushed out of the school system because of their inability to join online schooling. Those who have remained participants in digital classrooms have shown a distinct decline in cognitive skills. The dent in the education system is just one dimension of how children have been impacted. Even if they have been spared the worst medical manifestations of the virus, the invisible costs are almost more lethal and won't be fully known for years to come. Hundreds of thousands of children have lost one or both of their primary caregivers. Others have witnessed extreme trauma. A baby saw her mother die on a railway platform. Toddlers walked hundreds of kilometres home without food or water. And young girls are being forced into illegal underage marriages.

12

The Children of COVID

Some wore their hair short, cropped closely to their jawline, others pulled it back in ponytails that seemed to move in rhythm with the football. They all wore starched black shorts and deep-maroon T-shirts paired with socks that ran up to their knees to brace their bodies from frequent falls in the field. It was the sort of summer day when the desert heat forms a thick layer of smoke over the roads and the best hope you have of surviving it is to find a shady spot under a giant tree and sleep till it passes.

But not for these girls.

Most of them were between ten and seventeen – schoolgoing teenagers for whom sport was a much-needed escape. Even the shorts they wore that afternoon – something that other girls in the big cities can do without thinking twice – is a symbol of battle for them. It had taken argument, persuasion, pleading and fighting to be allowed to wear them instead of the more traditional salwar kurta.

As the girls kicked the ball around in the sand, their faces lit up with the sort of optimism that is the preserve of the young. Football had always been exhilarating for the hint of freedom it offered. Just imagining the possibility of an unchained life allowed them an escape into daydreams that the daily drudgery of their existence forbade.

But now, in the age of COVID-19, football had become more than about just aspiration. It was about guarding their childhood; it was about survival.

A maze of twists and turns through the Aravalli mountain range, now more shrubby than forested, had brought us to the village of Hansiyawas in Ajmer, Rajasthan. Barren and dusty, it lies huddled in an obscure nook several miles away from any urban pocket.

On the day of our visit, Sapna and Monica, sisters who are seventeen and fifteen, were fighting with their grand-uncle, village elder and patriarch of the family. Their brother's marriage had been fixed and the uncle argued that it would be financially smart to get the girls married off on the same day.

Sapna, with dreams of becoming a bureaucrat, and Monica, who thinks she might want to become a cop or play football professionally, had both managed to buy some time. Their weddings had been postponed, but their engagements stood intact, with boys they had never met, underage youngsters like themselves. 'I want to be known for myself, I want my identity to be defined by my work,' said Sapna, folding a pair of maroon football shorts fresh from a wash and iron. 'I do not want to be known by my husband or in-laws' name. *Shaadi* right now would be a *bandhan*, a chain.'

In all the grave ways Indian children have suffered through the pandemic, perhaps none is as calamitous as the increase in forced, illegal marriages, in particular the rising pressures on adolescent girls. Grassroots activists, who first brought football to rural Rajasthan in the hope that it would allow girls a larger window to the world, now believe the pandemic has set back their efforts by several years. In the summer months of June and July 2020, Childline, a hotline run by a government-affiliated agency, reported a 17 per cent increase in SOS calls related to forced marriages.[29] The number of complaints registered under the Prohibition of Child Marriage Act increased by 50 per cent in 2020 over 2019.[30]

'I cried a lot when they fixed my marriage,' said Monica, squatting on the floor and leaning against a pale white wall. 'I made my mother promise that she would find a way to stop it. It felt really strange – *ajeeb* – to be even talking about marriage when I have so much else to achieve.' Monica had never heard of football until the 'Didi' from the women's rights NGO introduced her to it; girls did not play any sports in Hansiyawas. And football, especially, was considered a boys' game. Monica and her friends began playing in salwar suits, a cotton dupatta tied across one shoulder and knotted at the waist, to reassure orthodox villagers that their modesty was intact. When they moved to wearing shorts, they wore leggings or trousers below so that their legs were not visible. Now they finally played in regular kit and gear, but it had taken a long time to get here.

'I want to play football for India,' said Monica. 'I do not want to get married at fifteen.'

India holds the ignominious distinction of being home to the largest number of child brides in the world, accounting for one third of the global figures. Every year, at least 1.5 million, or 27 per cent, of girls get married before they become adults. Staggering though these figures are, they actually reflect a downward curve. A decade ago, 47 per cent of Indian girls under eighteen were pushed into illegal unions.[31] The government has legislated to increase the legally permissible age for girls from eighteen to twenty-one, to make it the same as for boys. But a complex mix of economic factors, social prejudice – and now COVID – is reversing several of these gains.

Indira Pancholi sat under the shade of a tree with close to a hundred girls squatting cheerfully all around her. As long as the activist with the Mahila Adhikar Samiti, a women's rights forum, was distributing glucose biscuits and fist-sized packets of Lays chips, to be wolfed down with orange juice, the kids were giggling, chatting, whispering excitedly among themselves, as kids do. Then came the tough part. She had to draw them out on how many of them were under pressure to get married or engaged. Hands went up slowly, falteringly, one by one. Girls no older than ten or twelve, pint-sized child stars for their courage in the face of the bleakest of realities, raised their arms, but kept their eyes down in acknowledgement of the helplessness they felt.

Indira was now dealing with the most sensitive part of the dialogue: Has any girl been abused at home, faced violence or sexual abuse, she asked gently, her voice dropping to a whisper. A silence fell over the group; they huddled closer together. Their mothers had already been speaking to Indira and her team in confidence. The data too tells its own sordid tale. Lockdowns, restrictions on mobility and job losses have pushed men into long hours of confinement in tiny quarters, where there has been nothing separating them from their spouses or daughters. Pornography, masturbation, non-consensual sex with their wives while the children watched, and yes, violence ... this is what girls and their mothers have reported back to women's groups across the country, said Indira.

Customarily, after the marriage of a pre-adolescent girl, she continues to stay with her parents till the *gauna* ceremony, a send-away-to-in-laws date on the child marriage calendar, when the girl is considered old enough to have sex and consummate the union. Theoretically, this is when the girls start menstruating. But, as social awareness spread and girls began spending longer years in school, they would persuade their parents to let them stay on in the village at least till they turned eighteen.

The pandemic has upended that progress.

If it weren't the men of the village looking to save money with mass weddings, now mothers had increasingly begun to see the home as an unsafe space for their daughters.

'As girls began to complete education till class ten, they also began to dream,' said Pancholi. 'Someone wants to become a teacher, someone wants to join the IAS. Now, girls are giving up on their dreams again. Because schools are closed, girls are visible, hanging about in the village, and families say, if there's nothing else let's send them away. With men spending long hours at home, the space for girls has shrunk. Often the husband will have sex with his wife when he wants, whether she wishes to or not. Women are not able to stop their men or sons. They think their daughters will be safer elsewhere.'

And so, in the open-air class that day, Indira Pancholi introduced us to nine-year-olds and twelve-year-olds who are being asked to leave the village for their so-called husbands' homes.

Pancholi explained that when schools were functional and frequent shutdowns were not the norm, the girls could earn small money by running tuitions for younger kids, helping out at a local beauty parlour or spending a few hours chipping in at the neighbourhood *kirana* stores. This gave them a certain degree of autonomy and confidence. Now they feel their choices have shrunk.

If 2020, the first year of the pandemic, was about emotional and physical displacement for children as a result of the lockdown and the mass exodus of migrant workers; the second wave in 2021 brought home the lethal social and mental consequences for millions of Indian children, both urban and rural.

The physical closure of 1.5 million schools has impacted 247 million Indian children enrolled in elementary and secondary schools. Movie halls, malls, restaurants and gyms opened in India well before any attempt was made to restart schools.

Well before COVID, 6 million girls and boys were out of school. Now millions more have fallen out of the school system. On paper, online classes have continued. But the absence of equity in access to the internet, and to computers and smartphones has made the virtual school a horrifyingly unequal space. Only 24 per cent of India has access to the internet and just 11 per cent have computing devices.[32]

Even the matter of whether a child received basic learning material was impacted by whether he or she used a smartphone or not. Of children who had access to smartphones, 50 per cent were likely to receive learning material. Of those without one, this figure whittled down to a mere 17 per cent.[33]

The consequences have been even fatal.

In Shadnagar, a small town 50 kilometres from Hyderabad, the glitzy tech capital of India, Srinivas Reddy, an auto mechanic who in better times earned ₹400 a day, learnt this in the cruellest way possible. Srinivas and his wife Sumathi, who stitches clothes for a living, had to make a terribly difficult choice when it came to educating their daughters, and had prioritized one over the other. To educate their elder child, Aishwarya, who routinely aced exams at school, they were forced to stop sending her sister Vaishnavi to school. Aishwarya, with dreams of joining the civil service, stood second in the town in the class twelve board exams, with a score of over 98 per cent. Education offered her a glimpse into a world full of possibilities, but money was limited. Srinivas mortgaged his small house for a loan of ₹200,000, and his wife sold the little gold that she owned to send her to Delhi to enrol in the maths programme at Lady Shri Ram College. The younger daughter was pulled out from school after she completed her seventh grade so that the family could concentrate their resources on one child.

Today, their one-bedroom house, against which a pending loan still stands, is a shrine to nineteen-year-old Aishwarya. There are photographs of her everywhere – her jet-black waist-length hair worn straight, her pastel, lacy dresses that slowly made way for T-shirts, jeans and scarves as she got used to Delhi, pictures of her posing proudly at the Mughal Gardens in the Rashtrapati Bhawan and the Taj Mahal, smiling a toothy, hopeful smile in each one of them. In one corner of the room, Sumathi's sewing machine sits on a plain wooden platform. Scattered around her dead daughter's photographs are bits and bobs of coloured fabrics that she will tailor into kurtas and dresses; the steep 25 per cent interest on the loan they took to educate their child still remains to be paid.

In 2020, LSR, like every other institute, had gone online, terminating physical classes as India went into lockdown. Aishwarya was also asked to vacate the hostel room and head back home.

Once back came the challenge of how to study. Aishwarya needed a proper phone, Srinivas tells me, Vaishnavi flanking his side, her arm linked with his. 'I didn't have the money to buy her either a One Plus or a laptop. She slipped into depression.'

Srinivas saw Sonu Sood, an actor-samaritan on television who had become a national figure for his charity work during the pandemic, and reached out to him. But it was already too late.

On 2 November 2020, Aishwarya killed herself. 'If I can't study, I can't live,' she wrote in her suicide note. 'I have become a burden on my family."

'She used to tell me everything on her mind – Dad, should I do this, Dad, should I do that,' said Srinivas, in faltering Hindi. 'Why didn't she tell me this time?'

For upper-middle-class children, the absence of physical learning has led to an eruption of lifestyle diseases. A spike in obesity, cardio-respiratory fitness and diabetes has been directly linked to the increased screen time and long sedentary hours at a table. There has also been a distinct regression in learning skills, puncturing holes in the thesis that virtual education can be just as effective as face-to-face communication. A five-state survey found that within one year, 92 per cent of children lost one language ability across age groups, and 82 per cent of kids at least one mathematical skill. A closer look at just one state – Karnataka – revealed that the number of children enrolled in standard two who could not identify even numbers 1–9 doubled from 12.8 per cent to 25 per cent in 2020. And those who could not read the letters of the alphabet jumped from 19.1 per cent to 32.6 per cent in 2020.

In the village of Bhalokhara in Agra district of Uttar Pradesh, nine-year-old Kangan wanted me to know that she could recite the entire English alphabet from A to Z. Her face sparkled with the satisfaction of a job well done and a toothy smile that ran from ear to ear. Her mousy, light-brown hair fell to her shoulders, dancing in the wind, as she scampered through her village with her best friend, Khushi. In her arms, she cradled her infant brother at the same time.

The men of the village sat on their haunches, their dhotis pulled to their knees, as a herd of buffaloes nibbled at stacks of hay at the back. The women sat segregated in a different corner, their heads covered with the coloured edges of their saris.

The children often played by the village pond, nestled in the cool and serene shade of a natural canopy of trees. There I sat with the girls, marvelling at their magnetic energy and resilient good cheer.

There was a giant lock on the bright red door of the village *paathshala*, even though with its open grounds and airy rooms, it had enough cross-ventilation to make it safe to attend. The kids had started out delighted to have time off. Now they were being pulled into labour – working in the fields, shepherding cattle and fetching water.

'How do you pass the time?' I asked Kangan. 'In the evenings, I play. Otherwise, I do *jharoo-poncha* (sweeping and mopping).' As her baby brother sat in her lap and pulled at the strings of her yellow slip dress, she did not hesitate when I asked her what her dream was for the future. 'Mummy says, I must become a doctor. I like the idea too.'

Kangan and Khushi took us around the village school. On the corridor wall were two striking boards. One was a charter of children's rights; the other the meal menu for the week. Dal-chawal on Tuesdays, soyabean sabzi on Mondays, fruit on Saturdays.

As with everything else, the real story of COVID is the story of stark inequality. In the cities of India, the middle class and elite could afford to debate when exams should be held, whether school buses were safe and whether classrooms needed to be redesigned. But for millions of poor children, especially in rural India, not going to school meant something dire – going hungry. India's midday meal scheme, the world's largest mass-lunch programme, feeds 120 million children with one hot, healthy meal every day. Though the central government ordered that the food must continue to be available to children during the pandemic, states struggled to execute this. In the first two months of the national lockdown, 60,000 less tonnes of grain were lifted by state governments across India than is usual for the food programme.[34] Despite the government announcing a take-home-ration scheme to compensate for the closure, 35 per cent of schoolchildren did not receive their midday meals. Of the remaining 65 per cent, only 8 per cent received cooked food.[35]

COVID made India confront stark realities that otherwise remain buried in research papers, academic surveys or government files. The wide disparities that were only newspaper headlines to the privileged were the lived lives of the vast majority of the nation. And the pandemic compounded each such socio-economic imbalance.

Between rural and urban India, online schooling went down differently. Less than 15 per cent of India's rural population has access to the internet, against 42 per cent of urban homes. The discrimination does not end there. From food to phones, boys have been privileged, ahead of girls. A smartphone in the hands of a young girl has long been associated with unwanted autonomy, imagined sexual permissiveness and a secret world that resists control. This gender divide is reflected even in adult access to smartphones – women are 15 per cent less likely to own a mobile phone and 33 per cent less likely to use mobile internet services than men. In 2020, 25 per cent of the adult female population owned a smartphone, against 41 per cent of men.

As schools went online, households that had only one phone and a boy and a girl invariably allowed the boy to study ahead of the girl.

Sitting huddled together on a charpoy after a sweaty game of football, the girls of Hansiyawas village spoke of being denied the use of a smartphone at home.

This prejudice, they said, had created the perfect excuse for their parents to force them to get married. The pandemic years had not just taken away their right to education; they had underscored their status as children of a lesser god.

Pinky Gujar is fifteen and was engaged to be married at the peak of the COVID second wave at her grandfather's insistence. 'I felt I had been abandoned, I was so angry. I felt all alone,' she said, describing weeks of argument and resistance at home. 'No one stood with me.'

Finally, her father agreed that the engagement would not be accelerated into a marriage immediately. Pinky has never met or seen the boy she is meant to marry. 'I am not interested,' she said.

'People say that a husband is important for a woman. But I think a job is more important for a woman than anything else,' Pinky, so much older than her fifteen years, declared. She pointed in the direction of her friend Payal Prajawati, who was married when she was nine years old. Since the pandemic wrecked the social and economic equilibrium of life as they knew it, Payal's family has been asking her to go and live in her marital home, which is in a different village. Since the first lockdown, engagements are being accelerated into full-fledged marriages, Payal explained. In homes where there are daughters, parents are saying: whether you marry now or later you have to do it, so may as well do it now. '*Saste mein karna chahte hain.*' (They want to save their money.)

Many girls here have simply stopped attending online classes and are effectively no longer at school. 'Whenever they saw us with a phone they would accuse us of talking to boys,' said Payal.

'They took away our phones. Imagine, in our own village, this is how we are treated. Where there is one phone or just enough cash for a modest data plan, our parents have privileged their sons ahead of daughters. They get freedom, we get nothing.'

As we spoke to the young girls, we noticed another group of girls filming us, standing in a single row, aiming their smartphone cameras in our direction. The phones that their families won't let them have been provided to the girls by the same activists who introduced them to football. The aim is the same: to find ways to give voice, purpose and confidence to girls whose rights are being trampled upon, now even more than before. The phones were being used to train the girls in videography and journalism. For the vocational skills to eventually translate into autonomy, it was imperative that the girls weren't banished into enforced, underage illegal unions and had enough years to build capacity for economic self-reliance. Already, not going to school had hurt them, not just intellectually but in far more basic ways.

For the poor, schools in India are about so much more than what the classroom offers. From losing out on nutrition to sanitary pads, Indian girls have been the biggest victims of the shutdown.

The hesitation in opening schools, unlike in the West, is not just because of the sheer numbers of students crammed into single rooms, often in spaces with little ventilation; it is because of the continued, unresolved debate over how the virus impacts younger people. Scientists remained divided over the vaccination of children. A vaccine by Zydus was approved for emergency use in August 2021 but it was not till Christmas that year that the prime minister gave the green signal for older children to get the jab. Through the second wave, paediatricians argued that children had reacted differently to the Delta variant from the way they did to the first wave of COVID.

The SRCC Children's Hospital in Mumbai makes a real attempt to look friendly. Its exterior walls are made from rainbow-coloured panels, there are bursts of sunflower yellow in the nooks and crannies of its interiors and a spiderman right at the entrance. Murals of fairy tales run along the walls, a tortoise here, a rabbit there. There's even a miniature playground with swings and slides.

Inside the ICU, over the staccato beep of the machines that monitor vital signs – heartbeat, heart rate, body temperature – the soft cry of a newborn was clearly audible. She was wrapped in a candy-striped pink-and-green blanket. From under the fabric, her tiny hand stuck out, quivering every few seconds when the ventilator set off a tremor. It's a special kind of ventilator, Dr Soonu Udani, the medical director of the facility, explained, programmed to wiggle the body. The baby was eighteen days old and was fighting for her life.

Science is conclusive that the virus does not transmit internally from mother to child through the placenta. But babies can pick up the virus just the same way adults do, from close contact with an unmasked infected person in a space that is poorly ventilated. In fact, in the pandemic years, newborns had been especially at risk during hospital deliveries. And the delay in green-signalling vaccines for pregnant women meant new mothers who tested positive for COVID became a threat to their infants after they were born, often resulting in enforced separations between mother and child right after the delivery. Horizontal transmissions have been a severe challenge.

The eighteen-day-old infant was heavily oxygenated because the pneumonia was so severe it had burst a lung. She was ensnared by tubes that were bigger than her frame. The baby was brought to the speciality hospital from Nashik to Mumbai by road, her condition worsening on the way. A high-frequency oscillation machine had been deployed to try a different method of ventilating from what is used for adults.

Mumbai was riding the crest of the second wave in April 2021 and Maharashtra topped the charts with the highest number of COVID cases. Walking me through the COVID children's ward, Udani, a normally unruffled, cheerful Parsi doctor with decades of experience, was distinctly anxious. From her perch, at this inflection point in the history of the virus, things seemed very different from the first wave. 'In 2020 we put in protocols, we segregated the wards,' she said. 'But we had wasted capacity; we had more beds than we needed and we treated mostly everyone at home. This year it's different. Almost every child who has come to hospital is quite sick,' she sighed, pointing to at least five children who are on ventilator support. 'Last year, one out of 120 kids had bad pneumonia. This year that number has risen to five. Children are showing adult-like vulnerabilities; obesity, for instance, has become a comorbidity even among children, making overweight children especially vulnerable. This year we are in trouble.'

The hospital had to rewrite the COVID isolation rules that have typically kept families apart, with parents and children sometimes unable to meet even in their dying hours. Udani believed that children made for different patients and needed someone by their side. And so, by every bed in the ICU was an overanxious parent, trying to be more cheery than they felt, gently urging a child to allow the nurse to read her oxygen levels or measure her body temperature. By the side of some beds, exhausted mothers caught a catnap or a few moments of respite, slumped in the ward's white plastic chairs, grateful that the worst had passed.

Parents had come armed with colouring books and crayons and comics, and when all else failed there was always the phone. Mindless screen time, typically forbidden at home to kids, was encouraged as a happy distraction. This was COVID. None of the normal parenting rules applied.

In one alcove of the ICU, a child was pulling at her mother's mask, partly playful, partly agitated. When the attendant stopped by to place an oximeter to her finger, she pushed the cable away and burst into tears. Her mother bent down to whisper something softly into her ear in a calming but loving tone. The child quietened down, leaned forward, planted a kiss on her mum's lips and then clapped delightedly, her deep-black eyes suddenly twinkling.

Prarthana, sixteen years old, was a non-verbal special-needs child. Unable to speak in words, she communicates through gestures, sound and facial expressions. Her mother, Prety Kutty, had added a new word to their special grammar – mask-wala-kiss – to describe the kiss her daughter just gave her. Dressed in a block-print pyjama suit, short hair that fell in waves on her shoulders, Prarthana had bandages around her wrists and a cannula inserted in her hand, which was making her acutely uncomfortable. At first, she took out her irritation on Dr Udani by pressing her hand against her plastic PPE gown, as if to say go away, leave me alone. Udani lingered on patiently, allowing the mother to take the lead on how the nurses and doctors should intervene.

Prety told me that when Prarthana first tested positive the family found it impossible to get a bed for her. They lugged oxygen cylinders and concentrators home, but her vitals were borderline and precarious. She dialled every government hotline, but apparently no one among policymakers had paused to consider what may happen to children with special needs. 'All children, verbal and non-verbal, sometimes do not speak up when they are experiencing trauma,' she explained. 'Prarthana, being non-verbal, cannot tell us what she is feeling, and that is what makes this so tough. But that is when mothers have to step in.'

The disabled community may have been the most invisible group in the COVID crisis, children most so. For parents of special-needs children, a kid getting COVID is an all-consuming commitment. By December 2020, a rapid assessment across four states revealed that 77 per cent of parents of disabled children had lost their jobs.[36]

After the Delta variant gave rise to crowded ICUs in paediatric facilities in the second wave of the pandemic, state governments went into panic mode. Maharashtra's task force, for instance, controversially warned that when and if a third wave hit India, it could disproportionately affect children. The chief minister got on to a Zoom call to order the opening of special family hospitals across the state. Child specialists like Udani began advocating vaccines for children in order to be ready for what came next and also to enable the reopening of schools. Mumbai's dynamic municipal commissioner Iqbal Chahal made children's hospitals his priority and said doctors had advised him to prepare for a paediatric wave. At the time the belief was that as the virus mutated it was targeting younger and younger age groups. So, if the first assault of the virus had ravaged those above sixty years of age, the second appeared to hit those between eighteen and fifty. The next time could mean the nightmare of eighteen and younger facing its wrath.

But with time, and as the wounds of the second wave slowly began to turn to scabs, scientists were able to step back and make a more dispassionate assessment. In August, the National Institute of Disaster Management agreed that there was no medical basis to believe the next eruption of the virus would specifically target children. And global studies reaffirmed the finding that children were at minimal risk of severe illness. But nor was there any escaping the fact, the committee warned, that there was a severe shortage of paediatric infrastructure. Hospitals, ambulances and doctors would all run short if there were to be mass infection among children.

The lack of consensus among medical practitioners over exactly how much society should worry for its children has shadowed the reopening of schools. An alternative view remains to vaccinate as much of the adult population, especially teachers, as possible, and not get too anxious about asymptomatic infections among children. Even when state governments, buoyed by declining caseloads, ordered the reopening of schools, middle- and upper-middle-class parents have refused to send their kids to school. Many big city schools reopened to empty classrooms.

The creeping, insidious damage to children will be felt in multiple ways.

Well beyond the medical consequences of COVID, the emotional and mental scars may leave greater damage.

I think of Nitin, the nine-year-old I met in Bhiwandi, in Maharashtra, as he clambered on to a bus back home to Uttar Pradesh with his father, a carpenter and migrant worker from Azamgarh. Do you know what coronavirus is, I had asked him, almost playfully. 'Yes, it means, I do not get food. I have to go hungry.'

I remember meeting Pallavi, a young impish girl, on the highway between Pune and Hyderabad. Her family was lucky enough to get a ride in the back of a truck in which they were packed in with scores of other people, when rain came pouring down. We were on the road, and the thunder grunted and the lightning crackled as the wind lashed against our car windows. As we pulled to the side to let the storm pass, we saw a truck parked right in front of us. It's flap at the back was open and an elderly woman, Manglaben, wearing a printed pink sari was sitting inside, knees dangling down, surrounded by a posse of small children. In the corner away from the road, a group of men sat huddled together talking; another bunch was trying to cook dinner in the rain on a kerosene stove – a meal of millets and rice. One of the workers was disabled and had no hands. He stood in the rain and looked on at the passing traffic, the darkness of the night reflecting his state of mind. These were cow-dung handlers or gobar workers heading from Mumbai back to their village in Karnataka. The truck driver had agreed to give them a ride for only a small part of the way; otherwise they, including all the small children, had done the journey on foot. Pallavi, in a bright blue kurta with her hair braided neatly, spoke to us quite cheerfully about walking an entire day without any food after the anda bhurji they had packed from home was consumed. When I asked her what she would like to do or be when this awful moment passed, she told me, 'I want to help the poor.' How did she want to do that, I asked her. 'By distributing food to the hungry,' she said, on a day when she had barely got anything to eat.

And I thought of Rohan and Shobhan, brothers, the former still only seventeen years old, who lost both their parents to COVID in the first wave. Their mother, Baikali Malik, was a teacher who contracted COVID after she was deputed to distribute rations in a local school; their father, Dr Ripon Malik, was a doctor, a general physician. Rohan was still in school; his elder brother had just finished college.

The family used to live in an unremarkable housing society in the capital, where rows of identical homes camouflaged the very individual tales of tragedy.

Shobhan and Rohan's mother was discharged from GB Pant Hospital and sent home when she fell sick again after briefly looking like she was recovering. In that small window of time their father caught the infection too. As the boys rushed their mother to a different hospital, they returned home that night to find their father in a semi-conscious state.

'It is not about who will cook or how we will manage for money: it's about dealing with the biggest loss of our lives,' Shobhan told me, as we walked past cookie-cutter balconies from which curious, half-sympathetic neighbours stared down at us.

They took out their family album to show us photographs of when Baikali was a young mother and the boys were toddlers in her arms.

'I am a kid,' said Rohan. 'I am used to my mother doing everything for me. Everything in my daily life was looked after by her. Today I had to wear a T-shirt for my online class and I had no idea where it was. Usually, my mum would have organized it for me. It's these little, tiny things that hit me. I realized – no one is ever going to do that for me again.'

At the RML Hospital where their mother spent the last three days of her life, there were not enough ventilators. The doctors needed to intubate Baikali, by placing a tube down her throat into her windpipe so she could breathe more easily. After the pipes were placed, the pump to manually ventilate her was handed over to her sons. 'My brother pumped our mother for an hour,' said Rohan, trying to hold back his tears, uncomfortable with big displays of emotion, as young boys are often conditioned to be. 'When we turn the lights off every night, I can no longer sleep. That image keeps coming back to me.'

At least 150,000 children in India have now lost one parent to COVID; in many families this has been the primary caregiver. According to a *Lancet* study, there was an estimated 8.5-fold increase in new orphans in India, from over 5,000 as of March 2021, to more than 40,000 in April.

In a small village in Mandya, Karnataka, two daughters, both younger than ten, jumped into the back of an ambulance to accompany their mother on her desperate journey to find a hospital; they watched her die on the cold floor of a hospital that refused her a bed. In Bengaluru, a nine-year-old was told that her mother had gone to heaven to fight COVID with Goddess Durga after she died in the sixth month of her pregnancy.

In Bhopal, Vanisha Sharma, sixteen, was left to look after her younger brother, Vivan, who was just ten, after both parents died from the virus. A month later she topped her class ten exams, armed with the precocious wisdom that the pandemic has thrust upon young lives. 'When someone really leaves you, they never leave, do they?' she asked me, stoic in her strength and even managing to smile every now and then. 'I learnt that life is full of ups and downs. The trick is to enjoy the ups and have the courage to face the downs.'

Vanisha composed a poem as a eulogy to her father. It was called, 'I will be a strong girl, Daddy, without you . . .'

And in Mumbai, the eighteen-day-old baby fighting for life on a ventilator did not survive.

In the first ten days of 2022, there was a fourfold jump in the number of COVID cases in India. The country entered the third year of the pandemic, triggered by Omicron, the seventh variant of the virus. The numbers were threatening to be nothing short of calamitous in scale, but the virus appeared to have changed character, both in symptoms and lethality. The new wave called for a re-examination of old protocols, but concerns remained; the denominator was so huge that even a fraction of hospitalizations in percentage terms could topple the health system. Some of the interventions from a twice-bitten nation like India were much more sure-footed this time around. The Indian Council of Medical Research, New Delhi, advised home isolation and cautioned against indiscriminate use of drugs in stark contrast to the previous wave. Omicron was at our doorstep even before we were fully able to comprehend the lingering impact of the virus or what is called Long Covid. The only thing that could be said with any certainty in 2022 was that the idea of 'zero-COVID' was a giant myth. We would have to learn to live with, and despite, COVID.

13

And Then Came Omicron

At first, I waited for COVID to 'end' or at least subside before I wrote this book, thinking I would have a less dated and more rounded story to tell. Over time, I realized that was probably never going to happen, at least not in the near future of my lifetime. Of course, it will likely move soon from being pandemic to endemic, like so many other infectious diseases that are embedded into the backdrop of our everyday existence.

But the original idea that leaders of some countries had (China, New Zealand, Singapore, Australia) about eliminating COVID is entirely utopian. There will never be a zero-COVID world, not even if we hunker down, barricade up forever and live without the freedoms we cherish. And there is a deeper philosophical question here: is there any point in saving lives if the very idea of life itself is so diminished?

As I send this book to print, the seventh variant of the virus, Omicron, is galloping across the globe and in community transmission in most nations, including India.

It is, according to some studies, the second-most contagious virus in the world, only behind measles. It replicates in the human respiratory system seventy times quicker than Delta, is four times as infectious as the original virus and twice as much as Delta.[37]

The third wave won't be the last one either. So, Omicron has necessarily changed the way we measure, understand and fight COVID. Case infections are spiking, but they can no longer remain what we look for on the dashboard; instead, going forward, our success in fighting this virus will have to be measured against hospitalizations and fatalities. Of course, if even a small percentage of a giant caseload ends up in hospital, it can overwhelm health systems, especially if a significant number of health workers are among those infected and forced to isolate.

But there is enough in the initial research that is hopeful. Omicron, by all accounts, is distinctly more contagious than Delta but also significantly less virulent.[38] Among the vaccinated, globally, most infections have been manageable at home. A majority of those needing hospitalization are the unvaccinated. It doesn't appear to be hitting the respiratory system either; the infected are not reporting plummeting oxygen levels or difficulty in breathing.

The best news is evidence that Omicron infections are providing a layer of immunity against the much more lethal strain of Delta.

And so, though 2022 feels like déjà vu, it does not have to be. Both preventive measures, like vaccines, and therapeutic measures, such as antiviral tablets, are now available, compared to where the world was at the end of 2020. Yes, much has been said about how Omicron can 'escape' vaccines after two shots, but it is important to understand that vaccines were developed primarily to guard against serious disease and death. And as long as they continue to do that, they are doing their job. Boosters will add the much-needed layer of protection.

But despite the fact that we have so much more knowledge of how the virus spreads – primarily in indoor, congested, unventilated spaces – and what we should be doing to fight it, what is perplexing and disappointing is how quickly we still move into the default position of panic and prejudice.

Angelique Coetzee, the South African doctor who first revealed Omicron to the world when she spotted it on a simple DIY rapid antigen test, showed exemplary transparency, as did her country with the rest of the world. Yet, several countries responded with ill-thought-out travel bans that Coetzee told me 'were nothing short of modern apartheid.' In Coetzee's experience as a practitioner, the humble Brufen 'worked like a bomb and vaccinated patients are recovering by day five or six on their own.'

In India, the first response to Omicron's rising cases by politicians was to announce 'night curfews', easily the most illogical and unintelligent response to the pandemic and designed to tick a theoretical box in their heads or create the illusion of action. Schools are once again in the crosshairs of this short-term thinking, even though our children simply cannot afford any more closures.

And once again, the first response of politicians displayed spectacular hypocrisy. Across parties, leaders stripped away economic and social rights from citizens, whilst addressing huge election gatherings, where people in the thousands were boarded into buses and trucks, often maskless, pushing against each other before being allowed entry into open maidans. As public anger has made itself felt and heard, the Election Commission, unlike during the second wave, has finally intervened to ban mass rallies. Most people think it is not enough. The wiser call – and one more consistent with other restrictions – would have been to postpone the elections entirely.

There is something egregious about the idea of closed schools and open polling booths.

My mind and heart race back to the hundreds of government employees forced into polling duty – and early death – at the onset of the second wave. I think of their families – the pregnant woman, the orphaned children, the ageing mother. Elections should have been the last priority.

Most disappointingly, instead of clear communication from governments and public figures urging people to isolate when they are able to and not seek panic hospitalization, we are back to resident associations 'sealing' buildings if even one case of Omicron is traced. Not only does this make COVID feel like a crime – all over again – and discourage most people from wanting to test, science tells you it is absolutely unnecessary. The stigma and fear that we had spent two years battling and defeating, by paying literally with the blood of those we love, has returned as if this were 2020 instead of 2022.

Of course, certain measures will always be essential. Masks may come to be a permanent and barely noticeable part of our landscape much as they are in Southeast Asia. A complete vaccine course may end up being even more than three shots, much like Israel, which is on its fourth. The COVID vaccine may even become an annual jab much like the flu shot.

To start with, vaccine passports should become as routine as using an identity card. Voices on the left and right of the aisle, depending on the country you are having the argument in, have claimed that this is coercive, illiberal and would hand over too much power to the state. But in fact, a vaccine passport may be the only counter we have against giving state's institutions sweeping powers to impose localized lockdowns, arbitrary curfews, curbs on education and an ad hoc shutdown of theatres, malls and gyms; not to mention the continued devastation for the economy and our mental and emotional well-being. It is much better, for instance, for a restaurant to ask for your proof of vaccination at the door than for the government to demand that it run at half its capacity and close earlier than normal. Played on repeat mode, the government-led approach of restrictions could effectively push the majority of small enterprises out of work and devastate the poor irrevocably.

That the vaccine-surplus Western nations have not been able to enforce rules on mandatory vaccines yet is nothing but criminal and callous self-indulgence. Mandates are never ideal, but when the choice is between enforcement and lives being wrecked, especially of those who live on the margins – which is precisely what would happen with prolonged curbs – they become the only ethical option.

COVID will not 'end' but perhaps 2022 might be the year that it pulls back far enough for us to see the world and ourselves more clearly than we can right now when it is right in our face.

It is in the pandemic's residue that the damage will linger.

Long Covid, for instance, remains officially unacknowledged in India and not fully understood around the world.

If there is one thing that I have heard over these pandemic years, from more people than I can count, it is this: 'I don't feel the same.'

Amit Thapar, 46, is tall, lithe and well-built. For his middle years, he is remarkably fit. An industrialist from Ludhiana, he was a regular half-marathoner and routinely swam 200 laps of a

25-metre pool before he got COVID. 'I thought I would be okay in just a snap. My fever never rose beyond 99.5. I didn't even have a respiratory problem. But I used to get a trembling sort of feeling, like a low current was passing through my body,' he told me. 'I used to walk 12 kilometres a day. Now, I can't even walk 2 kilometres. But I've gone into a cycle of weakness and fatigue. I am not the same person I was before COVID. And my doctors have no clear answers because all my blood reports come back normal. All I know is I desperately want my old life back.'

Jyoti Lavakare, an independent journalist, told me that for at least hundred days after she recovered from COVID, she felt 'tired even while resting.' Her blood pressure started fluctuating, her vision felt hazy and she felt she didn't remember things so well. Like so many of those who were over-pumped with steroids during the illness, she felt her weight rise and her joints swell. I went through exactly the same as her right after my bout of COVID and even ended up fracturing one ankle and tearing a ligament on the other after a simple fall on the reporting trail. I was told the prolonged use of steroids had lowered my immunity and weakened my bones.

For those of us who had COVID before Omicron, we still don't know what impact the combined tablets of zinc, ivermectin, vitamins, favipiravir, dexamethasone and azithromycin, the distinctly Indian cocktail of COVID drugs, had on us.

What part of what so many are struggling with months later is the virus? What part is the medication, and what part is severe mental stress?

India, like much of the world, is still in the process of comprehending what Long Covid will end up meaning for those of us who were infected. People have reported a variety of after-effects, from diminishing memory to hair loss.

Nutan Banga from Hyderabad's Indian Business School said she felt acute pain in her bones 'all the time.' She used to be able to complete reading a book in three days, but now, she told me, 'every few sentences I need a break, the restlessness is so severe, I can't even watch a movie at a stretch. Every time I tell someone about my hair loss, people turn around and say even cancer patients lose their hair. But it's not the same thing. We are not cancer patients. We had a flu-like thing that became severe, but we don't have cancer. Now I am scared to shampoo my hair. I am scared to run a comb through my hair.'

Scientists are now researching COVID beyond its respiratory impact; they are analysing its neurological consequences and impact on kidney function.

But certain manifestations of COVID have been mysteriously specific to India.

At the height of the second wave, in Bengaluru's HCG Hospital, an entire ward had to be staffed with specialist surgeons only to treat the curious spate of COVID cases compounded by mucormycosis or black fungus. Just in the span of a single fortnight in June 2021, fifty surgeries had been undertaken in this one hospital alone to remove tissues infected with mucor mold, usually in the eyes and nose and sometimes in the brain. There was still no consensus on whether the post-COVID phenomenon had been triggered by the overuse of steroids, by industrial oxygen or by the variant itself.

I met Laxminarayan, a sari seller from Andhra Pradesh, whose upper jaw and palate had to be surgically removed to contain the fungus. When he introduced himself to me, the words would no longer form; the doctors explained that after the operation, his nasal and oral cavities had merged, making routine bodily functions like speech impossible. Even swallowing, a mechanical, everyday involuntary action, would now be painful. But if the operation had not taken place, Laxminarayan would have died. He excitedly pulled out his phone and showed us the Andhra silks from the store in his village; he wanted to get back to work. The doctors were working on installing a dental prosthetic that would help him say a few basic words. He was excited to try it out, spelling the letters of his name phonetically, as if he had discovered it for the very first time.

The black fungus most commonly travelled from the sinus into the eyes; in many cases, the operations were, as one of the doctors said, 'removing an eye to save a life. It's about life over any other organ.' The accounts were horrific, and the affected patients were not so old either. The youngest person to be operated on for the mycosis was a twenty-one-year-old kabaddi player who recovered from COVID but ended up losing an eye to black fungus.

Radhakrishnan, a coconut farmer from a village 100 kilometres from Bengaluru started showing signs of the fungal infection fifteen days after he recovered from COVID. When I met him, there was a white gauze strip across the eye that doctors had just removed; the farmer, who was only fifty, almost the same age as me, leaned against a stack of pillows, in blue chequered hospital scrubs, staring out at anodyne white walls that he could no longer see clearly.

In the worst cases, like with Satish Kumar, the fungus had formed pus pockets in his brain. Kumar, a businessman from Andhra Pradesh only in his early thirties, was a father to a two-year-old. Doctors did not operate on his skull directly but went through the nose to the covering of the brain to remove his intracranial abscess. Now they could only pray that he would recover.

Like with everything else, the amphotericin injections, the most effective treatment, ran short. But they were also unaffordable for most poor patients. In Karnal, Haryana, I met the family of Rajwanti, a sixty-five-year-old woman from a low-income neighbourhood in the city, whose death was among the first recorded black fungus deaths in India. Her son, Rakesh, a stocky man who walked with a limp, held up a framed photograph of his mother, looking resplendent in a spring-yellow salwar kurta. He placed her portrait in the small outdoor verandah of his ground floor in front of two buffaloes grazing on a mound of hay.

The government medical college had asked Rakesh to organize the injections on his own, scrawling out the complicated name on a small piece of paper. Each dose cost ₹3,500, and she would need fourteen injections. This was after the family had already exhausted their savings on COVID treatment over twelve days. Rajwanti was diabetic, making her even more vulnerable to the steroids that had been used to treat her for COVID. Before Rajwanti died, her eye was infected with the fungus. 'We are daily wagers. Where are we expected to get the money from? The hospital only gave my mother a glucose drip. Everything else we bought.'

Black fungus has not been the only mystery, India-specific illness to erupt as an extension of COVID.

I also witnessed the phenomenon of 'bone death' or avascular necrosis. I spoke to Dr Vijay Deshpande as he lay propped up against a mountain of pillows on a hospital bed. He was still inspiringly cheerful. 'What's a hospital bed, when I have come back quite literally from a deathbed?' Deshpande, ironically an orthopaedic surgeon, was first diagnosed with COVID in 2020. Initially, he was treated with the usual cocktail of remdesivir and steroids; after eight days, tocilizumab was added as a disease modifier. He was placed in an isolation ICU alongside patients who needed kidney and heart transplants. 'Because of the heavy steroids and anti-coagulation pills, my right arm got swollen,' Deshpande told me. 'I underwent surgery on my right arm four times. My entire life depends on my right hand. I also need bi-dexterity. My left hand got weak, almost paralysed.' Deshpande's trauma did not end there. Between the first wave and the second wave, his left leg had to be treated for deep vein thrombosis, his left eye developed 'a throbbing pain and glaucoma because of the steroids' and he developed mouth thrush. 'I was about to die.'

Sanjay Agarwal, a Mumbai doctor, who researched the phenomenon of bone deaths during COVID called Deshpande's case 'the tip of the iceberg.' Doctors agreed that steroids were an effective life-saving intervention in extreme situations of the disease. But their use across the board had possibly endangered more than they had helped. Agarwal described the impact of what Deshpande and others were going through: 'Instead of being hard like wood, bones become soft like a boiled potato. The combined impact of the virus and possibly the steroids have lead to a blockage of blood supply.'

As Omicron cases spike exponentially, there is finally clear and unequivocal communication from many medical experts to not use any of the drugs that Indians were prescribed in the first phase of the pandemic. Lancelot Pinto, a doctor who was the first to call out the excess use of steroids for COVID treatment at a time when it was just not popular to say so, is warning against similar hasty shortcuts in the treatment of Omicron. This time around, India is witnessing the trend of well-heeled patients checking themselves into hospital to be administered with a cocktail of monoclonal antibodies. This is despite the fact that Omicron evades most of the antibody cocktails in use. A similar confusion surrounds the use of the antiviral drug molnupiravir, approved in India but not recommended. In the third year of COVID, the Indian Council of Medical Research has finally urged people not to self-medicate with remdesivir. I can't help thinking back to the number of desperate families I met who literally begged, borrowed and stole to purchase remdesivir and other untested therapies during the second wave. In 2018, roughly 55 million Indians were pushed into poverty because of out-of-pocket spending on health. It is hard to even contemplate what those numbers will look like in 2022.

On 5 January 2022, India announced the death of seventy-three-year-old Laxminarayan Nagar, the country's first Omicron-related death. Nagar suffered from both diabetes and hypertension.

It was on 10 March 2020 when the first COVID death from any strain was recorded in India. The person's name was Mohammed Husain Siddiqui, and he was seventy-six years old.

I returned to his family to understand where our journey through this pandemic began.

An eighty-five-foot-high statue of Lord Shiva towers over the Gulbarga highway that connects Hyderabad to the town now known as Kalaburagi in North Karnataka. The word in Kannada means 'stony land'. The sun was setting when I met Faisal Siddiqui, an Islamic scholar who lives in a pink-stone house with a shiny plaque nameplate nailed to its exterior. Faisal showed me the photographs of that fateful day that his father flew back from Saudi Arabia. The family went to receive him with flowers and bouquets. Ten days later he was dead.

'I don't know what happened. He had ice cream. Then he fell

ill,' Faisal's voice trailed off. He pored over his manual prime typewriter and from a bunch of plastic packets kept on the table beside it, he pulled out letters, documents, discharge slips and prescriptions. Faisal described what would become the all-too-familiar nightmare for Indians over the next two years – a desperate round of multiple hospitals to get his father treated.

In the nascent stages of the pandemic, only government-run hospitals and clinics were authorized to do COVID tests. The local clinic Faisal took his father to referred him to the Gandhi Hospital in Hyderabad. Hyderabad was more than four hours away by road, and night was falling. But the family clambered on to an ambulance and left.

In Hyderabad, Siddiqui's family went to three different medical facilities before one, a private centre, agreed to give him emergency care. But as his father's situation worsened, they discharged him saying they were not sanctioned to look after COVID patients. The family decided to return home. His father died on the way.

When I met Faisal Siddiqui, he did not want to believe that COVID had claimed his father's life. 'I have no paper that tells me he died from COVID. So, how do I know?'

From the early denialism of Siddiqui at a stage in the pandemic when the illness was still stigmatized, to a year later when families were desperate to be counted as COVID fatalities – in that ironic arc is India's COVID journey.

The third wave notwithstanding, we shall have to step out from the shadows of paranoia and fear into the sunlight of living again. COVID is here to stay as a fellow traveller on this journey. We can no longer wish it away; we can only manage it.

And if we have any respect for the two years of our lives that we lost – and for the people we lost along the way – all we can do is be respectful, empathetic and rational. We should listen to science, be sensitive to the gaping inequality all around us and mindful of our privilege, for those of us who enjoy it.

Across two summers, we have seen the virus expose all of our great divides. In 2021, the top 1 per cent of India earned 21.7 per cent of the national income while the bottom 50 per cent made just 13.1 per cent. The World Inequality Lab called us 'among the most unequal countries in the world.'[39]

As we rebuild ourselves from the debris of COVID, we would have learnt nothing if our hearts and minds are not moved by the staggering injustice of all that we saw.

In many ways, COVID, the contagion, is about the mystery and also the eventual miracle of science.

But if one were to ask me, COVID, above all, should be about a resetting of conscience, priorities and emotions.

As a nation. And as individuals.

The tryst with COVID is about us, we the people, the humans of this pandemic, the flesh and blood and tears and laughter that the data will never capture. In these strange times, so many of us have regressed into memories from our early years, looking for comfort in old familiars.

As I think of all the things I should have said to my father while he was still alive, I am haunted by the hum of one of my favourite tunes, a song from *The Muppet Movie*, a childhood staple, that suddenly seems to have new meaning about hope and optimism in midlife sullied by sorrow.

> Why are there so many
> Songs about rainbows
> And what's on the other side
> Rainbows are visions

But only illusions
And rainbows have nothing to hide
So we've been told and some choose to believe it
But I know they're wrong wait and see
Someday we'll find it
The Rainbow Connection
The lovers, the dreamers and me
Who said that every wish
Would be heard and answered
When wished on the morning star
Somebody thought of that
And someone believed it
Look what it's done so far
What's so amazing
That keeps us stargazing
And what do we think we might see
Someday we'll find it
That Rainbow Connection
The lovers the dreamers and me
All of us under its spell
We know that it's probably magic
Have you been half asleep
And have you heard voices
I've heard them calling my name
Is this the sweet sound that calls the young sailors
The voice might be one and the same
I've heard it too many times to ignore it
It's something that I'm supposed to be
Someday we'll find it
The Rainbow Connection
The lovers, the dreamers and me

Notes

1. 'Women and Water', National Commission for Women, January 2005.
2. 'State of Housing in India: A Statistical Compendium 2013, Ministry of Housing and Urban Poverty Alleviation National Buildings Organisation, Government of India.
3. Abhishek Dey, '2 MN without Ration Cards in Delhi Eligible for State Govt's Free Ration Scheme', *Hindustan Times*, 29 May 2021.
4. Report of the Economic Survey of Delhi, March 2021.
5. Data published by Ministry of Consumer Affairs, Food and Public Distribution, May and June 2020.
6. 'COVID-19 Livelihoods Survey: Compilation of Findings', Centre for Sustainable Employment, Azim Premji University, 2020.
7. 'Researching the Impact of the Pandemic on Internal Migrant Workers in India', United Nations Academic Impact (UNAI).
8. 'State of Working India 2021: One Year of Covid-19', Centre for Sustainable Development, Azim Premji University, August 2021.
9. 'Policing during India's COVID-19 Lockdown: A Review of Reported Accounts of Police Excesses', Commonwealth Human Rights Initiative, December 2020.

10. Public database of lockdown related deaths maintained by volunteers at https://thejeshgn.com/projects/covid19-india/non-virus-deaths/.
11. 'Rozgaar Survey Report: A Study on the Impact of COVID-19 on Migrant Workers in India', Daily Wage Worker Platform and Jindal Global University, March 2021.
12. 'Rozgaar Survey Report: A Study on the Impact of COVID-19 on Migrant Workers in India', Daily Wage Worker Platform and Jindal Global University, March 2021.
13. 'New Map Depicts 412 Acts of Pandemic-Related Violence and Threats to Health Workers and Services around the World in 2020', Safeguarding Health in Conflict, 3 February 2021.
14. 'Prachi Singh, Shamika Ravi and Sikim Chakraborty, 'COVID-19: Is India's Health Infrastructure Equipped to Handle an Epidemic?', The Brookings Institution, 24 March 2020.
15. Prashant Yadav, Abha Mehndiratta, Kalipso Chalkidou, Sidharth Rupani and Krishna Reddy, 'India's COVID-19 Testing Capacity Must Grow by a Factor of 10: Here's How that Can Happen', Center for Global Development, 1 June 2020.
16. 'Best Practices in the Performance of District Hospitals', NITI Aayog, Government of India, 2021.
17. 'Global Tuberculosis Report 2019', World Health Organization, 15 October 2019. Government response to starred question no. 178 in Lok Sabha on 27 November 2019.
18. Data published by Nikshay Portal, National Tuberculosis Elimination Program, Ministry of Health and Family Welfare.
19. 'Global Tuberculosis Report 2021', World Health Organization.
20. 'Impact of COVID-19 on Cancer Care in India: A Cohort Study', *The Lancet*, 1 July 2021.
21. Debasis Barik and Amit Thorat, 'Issues of Unequal Access to Public Health in India', *NCBI – PubMed Central*, 27 October 2015.

22. 'World Elder Abuse Awareness Day, 15th June, 2021: Human Rights of Elderly Are at Stake', Agewell Foundation, June 2021.
23. Government response to unstarred question no. 1687 in Rajya Sabha on 9 March 2021.
24. Chittaranjan Tembhekar, '"Citizens against COVID" Condemns Move by Cylinder Manufacturing Firms to Hike Rates of Empty Oxygen Cylinders', *The Times of India*, 11 May 2021.
25. Rhythma Kaul, 'Young Not More Prone to COVID-19 in 2nd Wave: Govt', *Hindustan Times*, 20 April 2021.
26. Amit Thadani, 'Preventing a Repeat of the COVID-19 Second-Wave Oxygen Crisis in India', Observer Research Foundation, June 2021.
27. Government response to unstarred question nos. 898 and 909 in Rajya Sabha on 27 July 2021.
28. Billy Perrigo, 'It Was Already Dangerous to Be Muslim in India. Then Came the Coronavirus', *Time*, 3 April 2020.
29. 'India's COVID Crisis Sees Rise in Child Marriage and Trafficking', BBC News, 18 September 2020.
30. Data published by National Crime Records Bureau.
31. 'Ending Child Marriage and Adolescent Empowerment', UNICEF India.
32. Data from 2017–2018 National Sample Survey Report on Education.
33. Data published by Annual Status of Education Report 2020 Wave 1 from the ASER Centre.
34. 'Food Grain Bulletin 2021', Department of Food and Public Distribution, Government of India.
35. 'Status Report – Government and Private Schools During Covid-19', Oxfam India, September 2020.
36. Nisha Vernekar and Pooja Pandey, 'COVID Caused 77% Parents of Disabled Children to Lose Jobs, 90% to Depend on Govt Support', *The Print*, 18 December 2020.

37. Hannah Devlin, 'Omicron found to grow 70 times faster than Delta in bronchial tissue', *The Guardian*, 15 December 2021.
38. 'Explained: Studies suggest why Omicron is less severe – it spares the lungs', *The Indian Express*, 3 January 2022.
39. Kiran Kabtta Somvanshi, 'India among the most unequal countries with an affluent elite: Report', *The Economic Times*, 8 December 2021.

Acknowledgements

If this book exists, it is because my editor and friend Chiki Sarkar did not give up on me. Through my frenzied journalistic commitments that took up nearly all of my time and my many phases of deep personal sorrow and debilitating depression, she was by turns gentle and firm. So, I owe her and the team at Juggernaut an enormous debt of thanks.

The idea of this book was born during the first wave when my father was still alive. I owe him more thanks than I can ever articulate. I have always been the person haring off into the great unknown, leaving my family behind for weeks on end and ignoring their anxieties about my well-being. Whether it was my reporting from war zones and conflict hotspots or my COVID reportage, over two decades, my father had to literally sit on his hands to cope with his fears and worries. Every time I travelled for work on a dangerous assignment, he would be unable to sleep at night, often yelling out loud from sudden short nightmares. But he never stopped me from pursuing my path. For the extraordinary freedom he gave me, one that defined me and made me who I am, I owe him eternal gratitude. It is because of that freedom and encouragement that I was able to travel across India for two years reporting on COVID.

To my team at Mojo Story, our digital media platform, that has held the fort so ably and brilliantly and allowed me the space to write this book, I owe more thanks than I can say. To the magically serene Shiralie Chaturvedi who single-handedly kept both work going and me calm and Zafar, Tarun, Ashish, Priyali, Mayank, Vinod, Vandana, Ritesh, as well as our entire team of camerapersons, social media managers, video editors, graphic designers, all our correspondents and colleagues – a special thank you, for the room to write this book and all the hard work on the ground that enabled it to begin with.

Thank you so much to Setu Loomba for the help with data inputs and research and for patiently absorbing the reality that my moods had more swings than the charts he had to study.

To the health workers of India, we owe special, unspeakable debt. Along the way, many doctors have come to be a part of my daily life and have counselled me and my family through all our trysts with COVID and more. For your generosity, help and public service, thank you. I am especially grateful to Doctors Ambrish Mithal, Harsh and Ritu Mahajan, Navin Dang, Ambarish Satwik, Ishwar and Trupti Gilada, Muffazal Lakdawala, Ritesh and Ravi Malik and Lancelot Pinto.

To all of you who showered me with food, clothes, help and love along the way, during my journeys on the road, even when you barely knew me or didn't know me at all, I am so grateful for the reminder that the human spirit shone through in the darkest times.

Finally, to the people of our country whom I have met and continue to meet in this third year of the pandemic – thank you for sharing your sorrow, deepest emotions and fears. Thank you for your fortitude, strength and, above all, hope, even in the bleakest moments. Thank you for trusting me to tell your stories.

Journalism is nothing if it is not about People First.

Thank you for reminding me why I became a journalist.

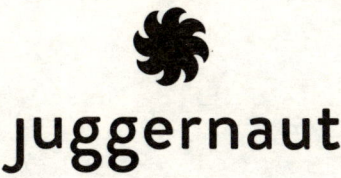

juggernaut

THE APP FOR INDIAN READERS

Fresh, original books tailored for mobile and for India. Starting at ₹10.

juggernaut.in

1

CRAFTED FOR MOBILE READING

Thought you would never read a book on mobile? Let us prove you wrong.

juggernaut.in

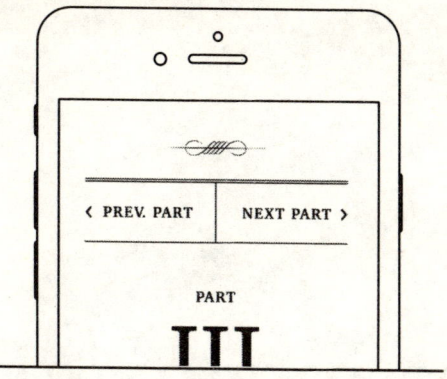

Beautiful Typography

The quality of print transferred to your mobile. Forget ugly PDFs.

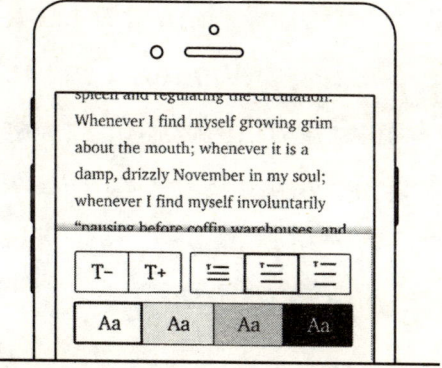

Customizable Reading

Read in the font size, spacing and background of your liking.

juggernaut.in

AN EXTENSIVE LIBRARY

Including fresh, new, original Juggernaut books from the likes of Sunny Leone, Praveen Swami, Husain Haqqani, Umera Ahmed, Rujuta Diwekar and lots more. Plus, books from partner publishers and loads of free classics. Whichever genre you like, there's a book waiting for you.

juggernaut.in

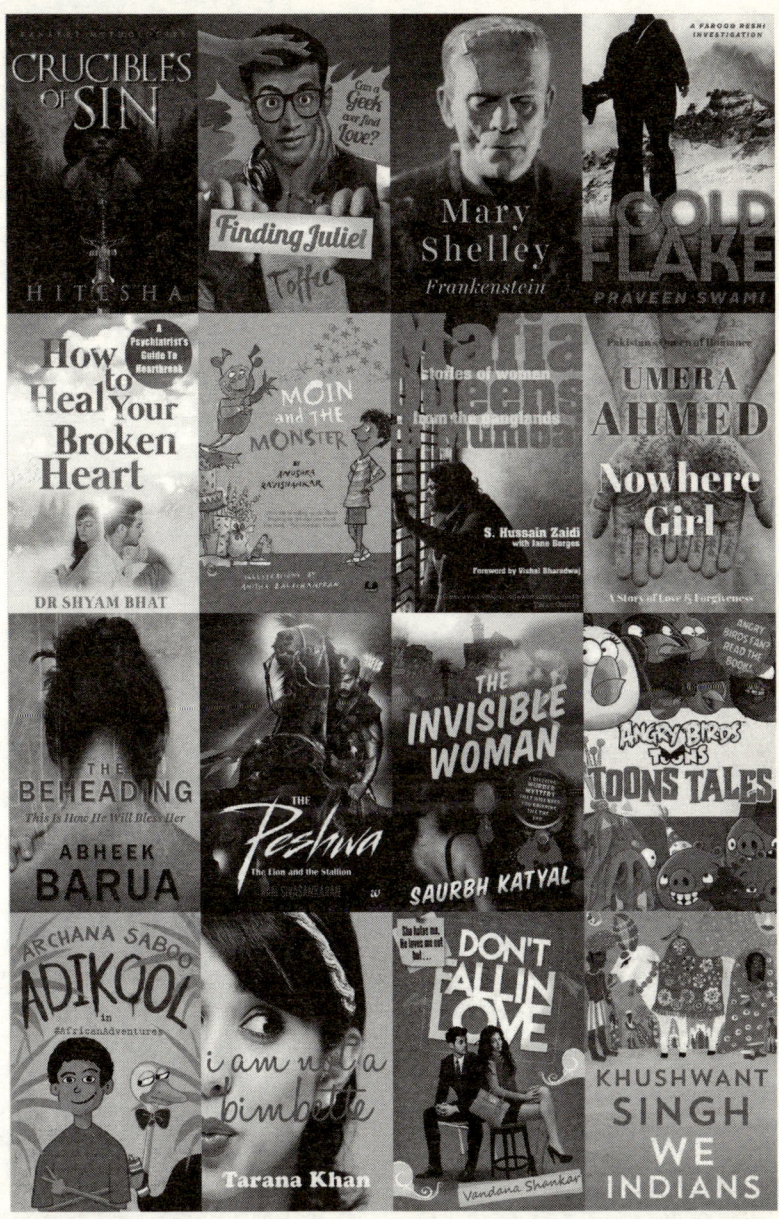

juggernaut.in

3

DON'T JUST READ; INTERACT

We're changing the reading experience from passive to active.

juggernaut.in

Ask authors questions

Get all your answers from the horse's mouth. Juggernaut authors actually reply to every question they can.

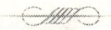

Rate and review

Let everyone know of your favourite reads or critique the finer points of a book – you will be heard in a community of like-minded readers.

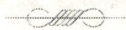

Gift books to friends

For a book-lover, there's no nicer gift than a book personally picked. You can even do it anonymously if you like.

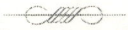

Enjoy new book formats

Discover serials released in parts over time, picture books including comics, and story-bundles at discounted rates. And coming soon, audiobooks.

juggernaut.in

4

LOWEST PRICES & ONE-TAP BUYING

Books start at ₹10 with regular discounts and free previews.

juggernaut.in

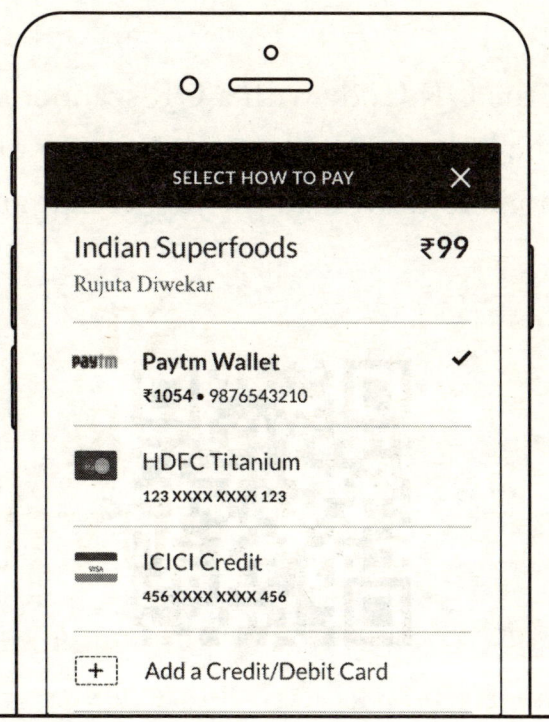

Paytm Wallet, Cards & Apple Payments

On Android, just add a Paytm Wallet once and buy any book with one tap. On iOS, pay with one tap with your iTunes-linked debit/credit card.

Click the QR Code with a QR scanner app or type the link into the Internet browser on your phone to download the Juggernaut app.

For our complete catalogue, visit www.juggernaut.in
To submit your book, send a synopsis and two sample chapters to books@juggernaut.in
For all other queries, write to contact@juggernaut.in